THE CORONA PROTOCOL — THREE —

SECRETS TO SUCCESS

PAUL D. CORONA, M.D.

The Corona Protocol

The Corona Protocol Three Secrets to Success
by Paul D. Corona, M.D.

Hardcover: 979-8-9998715-3-4
Paperback: 979-8-9998715-2-7
eBook: 979-8-9998715-4-1
LCCN: 2025923131
Published by The Corona Protocol,
30011 Ivy Glenn Dr., Suite 101, Laguna Niguel, CA 92677

www.drpaulcoronamd.com

Edited by Lisa Burnett
Cover Design: Jamie Simon
Author Photograph: Jackie Tran
Interior Design: Karen Corriente

First Printing Edition, 2026

Library of Congress Cataloguing-in-Publication
Corona, M.D., Paul D.
The Corona Protocol Three Secrets to Success
Paul D. Corona, M.D. p.192

ACKNOWLEDGMENTS

I want to thank my amazing assistant Leslie Perez, who goes above and beyond and is such a pleasure to work with every day in the office.

I want to acknowledge Lisa Burnett, who has not only edited these two books but also re-edited my first three books to be released as a second edition. I can't believe that she has never done professional book editing before, yet she has a gift for it. She is also my videographer for *The Dr. Paul Show* on Roku, Amazon Fire and YouTube. It has been a pleasure working with her on these projects.

Thank you to Karen Corriente for all her hard work doing the typesetting and layout not only for these two books but also for the second edition of my first three books *Healing the Mind and Body: The Trilogy.*

Thank you to Jaime Simon for the cover design of these two books as well as the second edition of my first three books.

Thank you to my patients who have taught me so much and have become friends. There is nothing I enjoy more than healing the minds and bodies of those that have entrusted me with their care.

Special thanks to my pastor, mentor and friend Chuck Smith Jr. who has helped me since the beginning of my writing journey 23 years ago. He has given me excellent advice and editing for most of my books.

Lastly I want to thank my father Arthur Corona, who has not only been incredibly supportive over the years but also has been a role model my whole life. Thank you to my wife Denise, my son Logan and my daughter Baylee. I also want to mention by best buddy and cat Seymour and our dog JG. I love you all very much.

TABLE OF CONTENTS

— SECRET #3 —

THE THREE SECRETS TO SUCCESS WITH THE CORONA PROTOCOL

My purpose in writing this book is to summarize the three areas regarding the treatment of mental health conditions that I strongly believe could be improved. Patients and providers need to recognize why treatment falls short for so many patients in desperate need of help. I realize that some of my views run contrary to modern opinions in this field of mind-body health, and my intention is not to complain or to be controversial, but rather I'm sharing my unique perspective about the subject.

Since I trained as a family physician I learned about the subject in a different way. I learned from the body to the mind, while psychiatrists learn from the brain/mind to the body. This is one reason why there are differences in perspective between our two specialties.

In over 33 years of clinical practice, I have developed these perspectives and opinions after a lot of practice with a lot of patients. I have certainly seen these three topics mentioned in psychiatric books and journals, but I am surprised about the lack of insight as to the importance of these areas. I have seen many patients who were previously evaluated by primary care providers as well as specialists and psychiatrists, and have observed their evaluations and treatment courses in order to try to understand and make sense of their perspectives, thoughts, and treatments. I would like to propose and introduce a different way of looking at things, and hopefully we can learn together and improve people's lives as much as possible, and over time be able to perfect the handcrafted cocktails, which are the building blocks of The Corona Protocol.

This protocol is all about optimizing the rational trial-and-error polypharmaceutical approach by balancing each neurochemical properly within the nervous system in order to perfectly balance the mind and body at the same time. This is the best tried-and-true method in order to assure the highest quality of life for each individual that we treat and care for.

I am purposely going to try to make this book as brief as possible while still being as complete as I need to be. I have addressed these topics in previous writings, but for this book I have distilled them down to the three most important topics that doctors need to learn. These issues are of such importance that they bear repeating. There are, of course, other areas and topics that are also important, but in the interest of time I narrowed them down to these *Three Secrets to Success*:

1) Recognizing that somatic symptoms relate to mood and that one necessarily affects the other.

2) Recognizing the full range of bipolar disorder, from the obvious to the more subtle variations of bipolar spectrum disorder.

3) Recognizing the importance of getting patients to achieve full remission.

SECRET #1

Recognizing that Somatic Symptoms Relate to Mood and that One Necessarily Affects the Other

SECRET #1

Recognizing that Somatic Symptoms Relate to Mood and that One Necessarily Affects the Other

The lack of recognition as to the importance of the mind-body connection is what really first grabbed my attention starting in my early years of clinical practice, and this topic then became the basis of what my first three books and other writings are about. By the end of medical school in the late 1980s, I was interested in several areas of medicine, especially internal (adult) medicine, pediatrics, OB/Gyn, and psychiatry. I ended up deciding on a three-year residency program in Family Practice in downtown Los Angeles, since I felt that being a family doctor would allow me to treat a broad range of patients and provide the most variety and the most well-rounded education in treating the whole person, or so I thought at the time.

I never seriously considered applying for a residency program in psychiatry, since I really didn't want to do that full-time. Looking back, I know I made the right decision, since otherwise I would not have discovered the incredible insights that I have had in order to be able to share this information with others.

I was certainly fascinated by my psychiatry rotations during medical school and during my residency program. On a rotation in a closed ward of a psychiatric hospital I was exposed to patients with schizophrenia and bipolar disorder with psychotic features, and I was fascinated by this. I wondered, "How can the mind become so ill in order to lead to these tragic consequences?" As I said, I didn't seriously consider during training treating this full-time, though I was already interested in mood and emotion, especially how this affects the person in other ways.

During my family practice residency program, I will never forget when one of the attending physicians told me, "Paul, at least half of what you will see in practice is stress-related." I started noticing how true that statement really was, though I found out that he underestimated. The majority of what we see in primary care is due to the interplay between the body and the mind. The two cannot be separated.

During my early years of practice and since then, I have witnessed a lot of common symptoms and diagnoses that are difficult to ascertain whether they are more mental or more physical. The reality is that there is probably a combination of both going on at the same time. These include:

- Neck/Trapezius/Upper back inflammation/spasm/ pain (probably #1)
- Headaches (muscular/tension, migraine, or mixed)
- Bruxism/TMJ inflammation and pain/Jaw clenching/ teeth grinding

- Lower back and mid-back spasm/inflammation/pain
- Fibromyalgia (scattered joint and muscular inflammation and pain)
- Fatigue (chronic and/or acute)
- Insomnia (difficulty falling asleep/shutting the brain down and/or early-morning awakening/difficulty getting back to sleep, or a combination thereof)
- Stomach problems such as acid reflux and peptic ulcers, dysphagia
- Irritable Bowel Syndrome (bloating, cramping, diarrhea, constipation, etc.)
- Dyspnea (shortness of breath, difficulty breathing)
- Excessive sweating
- Shakiness/Jitteriness
- Palpitations/Racing heart
- Hypertension
- Chest pain (inflammatory, costochondritis, etc.)
- Dizziness/Vertigo
- Skin symptoms (itching, rashes, infectious outbreaks, etc.)
- Chronic recurring bladder and urinary tract issues
- Recurring infections
- Hormonal symptoms such as PMDD/PMS, dysmenorrhea/excessive menstrual pain, menopausal

symptoms (pre-, peri-, and post-), postpartum, puberty, etc.

- Metabolic problems such as obesity, difficulty losing weight, difficulty gaining weight, etc.
- Chronic and/or Acute Whatever

In a primary care practice, we see such a variety of symptoms and medical problems, and it can be challenging at times to figure out what is being caused by what. Is it a “real” medical problem, or is it due to real stress and underlying mood? Is it both? This variety is what makes this job both interesting and fun. It’s like putting together a very interesting and intricate human puzzle, which, when completed and properly solved, has a major impact on the lives of those we serve.

I have observed that the usual treatment for these symptoms consists of symptomatic treatment such as pain pills (opiates and non-opioid analgesics), acid reflux medications such as antacids, H2 blockers, and PPIs that reduce heartburn fueled by stress, anti-inflammatories, muscle relaxants, sleeping pills, tranquilizers such as benzodiazepines, barbiturates, antidiarrheal medications, laxatives, steroids, steroid creams, inhalers, beta blockers, antihypertensive medications, stimulants, weight loss medications, dizziness/vertigo medications, etc. This is the way that physicians have treated such a variety of problems with so many “Band-aid” remedies that treat the symptoms after the fact rather than preventing them before they even occur in the first place. This is not to say that these types of treatments are not needed at all, but rather not as often. If we focus on prevention and not just reaction, this is a much healthier response, which leads to the best results.

In my humble opinion, this is not the way it’s supposed to be done. We can do way better by learning together. A much better way of going about it is getting to the root of the problem and treating it at its core. We have the pleasure of doing this with the best preventative and nonaddictive choices, which just happen to be psychotropic medications, which only balance neurochemicals if they are in need of being balanced in the first place. They only fix the problem if neurochemical imbalances are the cause, which is much more likely the norm than the exception.

The Corona Protocol is the most cutting-edge way to treat mind-body imbalances. It typically takes the right cocktails, which are figured out during the office visits and in-between by phone or email, in order to fine-tune the medications, which produces the most complete and satisfying results, with full and complete remission always the ultimate goal to achieve for all of those that we care for.

The root of the problem is not always what we can touch, test, and see with the naked eye, but rather has to do with emotion, mood, and attitude. As I said before, once I realized during training that the majority of what we see in the office is stress-related, then I was looking out for anxiety disorders, major depressive disorder, bipolar disorders, ADD/ADHD, etc. I found that stress and abnormal changes in mood correlated with some or all of the symptoms and medical problems that I listed previously. I started noticing that patients with unexplainable somatic symptoms also had an underlying diagnosable mood disorder the vast majority of the time.

Most of them, I noticed, didn't come in describing anxiety and abnormal mood but rather were focusing on their physical symptoms instead. I had to learn to explore beneath the surface and see what lies under the hood. We need to learn how to resolve the true underlying causes and treat them in the best preventative and healing way. It's always better to prevent problems rather than just dealing with them after the fact. Psychotropic medications are the healthiest holistic choices that help the body actually heal itself and achieve optimal mind-body harmony that we all should be able to achieve.

Initially during my residency training I was focusing primarily on symptomatic treatment, as I was trained to do and as I saw other doctors doing. However, once I started seeing what the real underlying problems were that were far more important than just the symptoms that were presented, I started shifting my focus regarding evaluation and treatment to a preventative treatment approach rather than a reactive one. After I finished my residency training in downtown Los Angeles in 1992, I moved to South Orange County to continue practicing what I had learned.

I really enjoyed being a primary care doctor, treating a variety of problems, which is what attracted me to the specialty of family practice in the first place. I also enjoyed developing personal relationships with my patients, treating them like friends and not just clients. I enjoyed (and still do) getting to know families and learning about what matters to them in their lives. I also was interested though, in the emotional and mental aspects of their situations after I understood that you can't separate the emotional from the physical since they are so intertwined.

My first exposure to the subject of human emotion was during my freshman year of college at USC when I took an Introduction to Psychology class, and I discovered that understanding emotion and why we behave as we do was fascinating to me and, in a sense, a "soft" science, which was a good complement to the "hard" science I learned as a Biology major. My increased interest in this subject was further fostered by my psychiatric rotations during medical school. As I said, I really did not consider a practice focusing on mental illness, as I have already done for over two decades, because I was also interested in the physical aspects of health. I knew that being a family doctor allowed me the opportunity to treat mood disorders as well as other physical problems. I figured out early on that following this unique path would be a unique opportunity and provide me the best of both worlds.

In actuality, primary care providers treat the vast majority of mental illness in our country. There are a lot more family physicians than there are psychiatrists, and there are not nearly enough psychiatrists to treat everyone who needs such treatment. Also, patients feel more comfortable being treated by their primary care provider that they know and trust rather than a doctor they don't know as well. They also may be hesitant to see a psychiatrist due to stigma, cost, availability, and other factors.

Primary care doctors as well as mid-level practitioners such as PAs (physician assistants) and NPs (nurse practitioners) are on the front line, and we are in the perfect position to be able to treat the vast majority of mind-body imbalances, since we learn a lot about the body and can see how it interacts with the mind. Psychiatrists can then focus on the more severe cases, such as those requiring hospitalization, those with schizophrenia or severe bipolar disorder, patients needing special types of psychotherapy for which they have been trained, and others who are at higher risk. However, there are some primary care doctors with significant experience treating mood disorders that feel very comfortable treating higher-risk patients. The truth is that I actually really enjoy the challenge.

I started treating depression and anxiety disorders during residency training and then continued to do so more and more once I started private practice. At that time in the mid-to-late 1980s and early 1990s, there were three "modern" antidepressants after the tricyclic antidepressants and the MAO inhibitors. These first three antidepressants released in this order were Prozac (fluoxetine), Zoloft (sertraline), and Paxil (paroxetine). I saw some very good results at times with some but not so good with others. I found that Prozac (fluoxetine) was very effective with certain patients, though sometimes it was too activating, made certain patients worse, and some had good results but also had bothersome side effects such as apathy, fatigue, sexual side effects, and others. Some felt better initially and then "pooped out" or got worse.

The second one, Zoloft (sertraline), seemed to have similar efficacy as Prozac (fluoxetine), and since it was a bit gentler, it was better tolerated by some, but still, in some, it tended to have the same side effect issues. I did not use the third SSRI, Paxil (paroxetine), as often. It had good efficacy for some with more agitated and anxious depression, but it was too potent for some, with a higher incidence of fatigue, weight gain, apathy, sexual side effects, the "SSRI poop-out syndrome" (which can happen with all in this class), and others. It's also the most difficult antidepressant to get off of, with an increased risk of withdrawal effects, which are not pleasant to experience and are best to avoid.

SNRI's To The Rescue

The big breakthrough came a year or so after I started private practice when Effexor XR (venlafaxine ER) came out. The first Effexor, prior to the release of the extended-release version, had a fairly high rate of nausea and needed to be taken twice a day with food, so I didn't initially see the benefit of this medication over the previous class, which was once a day and more convenient. It was initially referred to as "side-Effexor," which was why it was so nice when Effexor XR (venlafaxine ER) came out. Though some did not tolerate it, and in others it made them worse, as was the case with the SSRIs, more often than not they did quite well and tolerated it well. I started noticing that the efficacy seemed to be better overall than what I was seeing with the first three SSRIs, and certain side effects were absent or were not as bad as the previous ones.

I consider the SNRI Effexor XR (venlafaxine ER) the first "modern" dual-action antidepressant (since the tricyclic antidepressants and MAOIs work on more than just serotonin). These older classes though, had significant side effect issues, so I was reserving these for more complicated cases, which are rare. Effexor XR (venlafaxine ER) still had some significant side effects for some, such as activation, dry mouth, and nausea, though it had fewer sexual side effects and less of a chance of the "Poop-Out Phenomenon" as compared to the SSRIs. It is also second to Paxil (paroxetine) regarding difficulty getting off of it with withdrawal effects. It was quite clear to me though, that it was overall better for more people than the previous SSRIs.

Despite certain problems for some patients with Effexor XR (venlafaxine ER) at that time, overall, I was very happy with its efficacy and tolerance. I was noticing that the tolerability and efficacy were very good at the lower doses, but that the side effects increased as the dose was raised, and the efficacy, I discovered, was not necessarily better at the higher dosage range for many patients. At the time its manufacturer, Wyeth, while marketing the product, told us that it needed to be titrated up to the higher dosage range of 150 to 225 to 300 mg per day in order to achieve the best efficacy. They explained that it was even more noradrenergic and even dopaminergic at the higher levels.

I found in practice though, that this was true for some patients, but that most patients got very good efficacy and good tolerance at the lower dosage range while getting more side effects and not necessarily more benefits at the higher dosage range. I was wondering at that time why they were recommending this when I was having a completely different experience with it.

I was noticing that the efficacy of Effexor XR (venlafaxine ER) was faster than the SSRIs, and I was seeing surprisingly good results with the starter pack that provided the first week of the 37.5 mg capsule and the second week the 75 mg capsule. They then suggested increasing it to 150 mg, which they also sampled, since, as I said, the word was that the efficacy was better at that dose and above, reportedly even better at the 225 mg to 300 mg level. What I discovered though, was that excellent efficacy was seen at the 75 mg level and sometimes even at the 37.5 mg dose, and that more often than not increasing to 150 mg was too much.

I also found that in some patients the 37.5 mg during the first week provides excellent results and that increasing to 75 mg was too much with more side effects than benefits. Even though 75 mg is the most common dose, I had found that 37.5 mg was the second-best dose and that 150 mg was the third-best dose for the average person, with 225 mg in fourth place and 300 mg in fifth place. I've seen some doctors increase it to 450 mg or more, though I don't do that. This flew in the face of what the company was telling us, and I was curious and determined to find out why.

The company said that it was really no different than an SSRI at the lower doses, especially the 37.5 mg and even the 75 mg doses, but that was clearly not true. They were saying that we needed to get higher to get to the noradrenergic effect and even a dopaminergic effect at the highest dosage range. As I said, I typically find adequate noradrenergic and even some dopaminergic balancing at lower doses, but if more of a dopaminergic effect is needed, then I would more likely augment with the nDRI Wellbutrin XL.

I was curious at the time as to why the message that the company put forward was not the reality that I was seeing. I was noticing the positive noradrenergic effects even at the lowest doses since I was seeing resolution of somatic symptoms that I wasn't often seeing with the SSRIs.

As I just alluded to, the top augmentation strategy that I have employed is adding Wellbutrin XL. This is more dopaminergic than noradrenergic, though the slight noradrenergic effect leads to better efficacy if more norepinephrine is needed, though its main function is the excellent reuptake inhibition of dopamine, leading to a powerful dopaminergic and weaker noradrenergic boost that seems to fit quite well with SNRIs much more often than not.

It's important to start with the best initial medication in order to create the best foundation when it comes to augmentation and the rational polypharmaceutical approach. Wellbutrin is also a good augmenting step with SSRIs, but the increased noradrenergic focus with the "Dynamic Duo" of an SNRI with Wellbutrin XL more often than not leads to better and more complete overall results than an SSRI with Wellbutrin, though that combination also works well for many, which would be when norepinephrine is not a significant factor.

If we are not sure, then it is best to try both by comparing them back-to-back and seeing the results firsthand. There is no better way than witnessing and experiencing results firsthand with our patients. It doesn't get any better than that when it comes to clinical practice, which means practicing until we get it right.

As I said, I was curious as to why the company and representatives for Effexor XR (venlafaxine ER), as well as other doctors, were not understanding the simple message that it is usually better lower than higher. When I asked them that question and shared my own personal experiences with this product, they seemed confused, which confused me. Why weren't they seeing what I was seeing? The answer was that they weren't looking close enough at the details when the medication was titrated the first couple of weeks. The reason that they marketed it with the "higher the better" message was because that was how the product was studied and that was how the clinical trials were set up. Once they get approval, they can't veer from their original message. I wish they initially had studied it more at lower doses since that may have changed everything. This could have prevented the fatal error of their initial marketing strategy.

When doctors were dosing it too aggressively, they started seeing side effects that concerned them and scared them away because it would become too activating, which means feeling jittery or nervous with too much energy that doesn't feel natural. Doctors mistakenly thought that this meant there was an increase of anxiety, though this was often just a temporary side effect that the patient could adjust to. It could also mean that the dose is too high and needs to be adjusted down or that the titration needs to be slowed down. However, if it is significant in the person and if the person does not quickly adjust, then this is a signal that norepinephrine is not a significant factor and that this is not the correct medication for that individual. It may mean that an SSRI is a better choice.

There were also fears that it would increase blood pressure, though I recall a study that showed that this happened only very rarely, about 3% of the time. In reality, what I was witnessing was that it was actually more often decreasing the blood pressure. This made sense to me since when a medication reduces anxiety and stress and improves overall mood, this can also lead to normalization of blood pressure and other vital signs.

The result that I witnessed with this medication was truly amazing to behold. I couldn't believe what I was seeing so consistently. As I said, some referred to it as "side-Effexor," so because of this misperception, doctors have not changed their SSRI-first mentality even after all these years since then. We lost a valuable opportunity, since we could have and should have learned so much more by now.

The initial activation for someone when balancing norepinephrine usually goes away, and it is more calming than activating in the end, though in some it is energizing, so the hope is that it gives whatever is needed in each individual in order to balance the imbalances in the correct way. It was obvious to me in the early 1990s that Effexor XR (venlafaxine ER) was usually better than SSRIs, but I was still confused as to why other doctors were not catching on to this vital information. At first, I thought maybe it was just a fluke, but then I discovered it happened too often to be a fluke. I saw that what I was seeing was all too real.

What fascinated me most about the dual-action reuptake inhibitor was not only the improvement of depression, reduction of anxiety, and overall better mood, but also that I was seeing physical symptoms reducing, symptoms that I saw were stress-related. When I really started understanding the mind-body connection and what that really meant, I also noticed that mood is not only emotional and mental but also medical and physical. What surprised me was the amount and frequency of symptoms that I discovered were related to emotions.

That early recognition was what changed the direction of my practice then and thereafter. I started paying more attention to all the different physical/somatic symptoms that I was seeing improved when I would treat the underlying mood component. I discovered that the emotional and mood component was the true main underlying reason for the physical symptoms, and this message of treating preventively and not just reactively set me on the course that I continue to follow. It's simply just better to treat underlying problems earlier rather than waiting to treat them after the fact. I have found that it's difficult to treat the mind and body separately, since they're so interconnected, with one necessarily affecting the other.

I was surprised when I went to the initial lectures by doctors about Effexor XR (venlafaxine ER) that I was not hearing from them what I was learning about this product. Even when I went to a speaker training conference before I started lecturing to other doctors about this product, I was exposed to the same messages that I had previously heard, and even when I pointed out what I was learning already by using it, this still seemed to fall on deaf ears. Other doctors I spoke to didn't seem to understand that the best results are at the lowest doses and that there was significant somatic symptom reduction as well as excellent anxiety reduction and overall mood improvement at the same time. I shared with other doctors and company representatives that I was also noticing that it not only helped with depressive symptoms but also helped with symptoms of anxiety, which is more common and sometimes more impactful than depression.

I was noticing during training and early practice that these physical symptoms that I listed earlier in this chapter were so common. In many cases the symptoms were not the reason that they were coming in to see me, but when I teased out all of the pertinent symptoms, I realized why the patient was really here. They were coming in because they were just not feeling well, and I was noticing that they not only had physical/somatic symptoms but also significant stress and emotional problems. The more the stress, the more the symptoms. The more the symptoms, the more the person gets stressed out about the symptoms, which then leads to more symptoms, creating a vicious cycle that can be difficult to break.

As I said, I was initially confused by why other doctors I was talking to were not aware of the power of this message, but as time has passed, I have understood why this information is not more widespread. I was also initially confused as to why the pharmaceutical company that was making Effexor XR (venlafaxine ER) did not really reveal the improvement of somatic symptoms, further reduction of anxiety symptoms, and better improvement of depressive symptoms. I then figured out that one of the reasons was that they studied Effexor XR (venlafaxine ER) for major depressive disorder, so that was really all that they could talk about when promoting it. They could not comment about any other benefits, and if they were caught doing so, they could get into big trouble.

I asked many questions when I was training to be a speaker for the company, but when I spoke with the representatives and their managers, the only answer they could give was that they couldn't talk about it. When I shared my experience with the product, they didn't seem all that surprised, since I'm sure they had heard that before but realized that they really couldn't bring it up.

I spoke with other speakers who understood that it did more than just treat depression but were forbidden to discuss "off-label" benefits. "Off-label" means using a medication for an indication that it was not originally marketed for or that is not officially approved by the FDA and other governing bodies.

I have sat through many compliance lectures, usually by attorneys, at each of the multiple speaker training conferences that I have gone to, since I have been going to several speaker training conferences in order to speak about several different psychotropic medications. They told us what we could and couldn't say. They presented the "approved" slide deck and instructed us how to give the lectures, basically telling us to stick to the script. I did my best to try to get the message out as to all the benefits seen without crossing the line too much. It was important for me to try to explain to doctors what made each medication different and the many ways that it can be used.

"Off-label" benefits far exceed the "on-label" benefits of not only Effexor XR (venlafaxine ER), but also all the medications that came out before and after it. Depression only scratches the surface as to what antidepressants can be used for. I did as much as I could during the actual lectures to provide the most key information however I could and not just read the slides to them since I figured they could read them for themselves.

I had better opportunities to get my message across during the Q&A portion, my favorite part, as long as I pointed out to the doctors that I would be discussing "off-label" benefits that were not officially condoned by the manufacturer but rather my own experiences with prescribing it. They then became stricter as the years passed. They warned us to not solicit off-label questions, and if one was asked, then I was allowed to speak separately to that doctor after the lecture so as to not subject the other doctors to "off-label" information. I'm not kidding. I wish I were. I was amazed at the lengths that the FDA would go to in order to suppress off-label information. I just kept trying to get the word out the best that I could in order to educate doctors about the vital importance of this topic in the primary care setting.

I discovered that there is no such thing as free speech in medicine when it comes to discussion of medications and their uses in the public sector, though thankfully I have the freedom of speech afforded by the First Amendment when it is between myself and patients at the office or when I'm writing or speaking, as long as it is not sponsored by a pharmaceutical company. I initially wondered why the FDA and federal government were so threatened by the discussion of off-label benefits. Did they not see that off-label treatment means the most cutting-edge treatment? I wondered why they felt so threatened by the concept.

What I found out was that the biggest reason was that this is a good way for them to make money, a lot of it. If a company, sales representative, or doctor who works for them by speaking is caught implying promotion of off-label benefits, that company gets fined an excessive amount of money. Many pharmaceutical companies have had to make large payouts for this reason. There is a financial incentive for the government to find reasons to fault a company for perceived violations. This scares companies into making sure that this cutting-edge information does not get to the prescribing doctor.

The big problem, though, is that the majority of doctors never hear this information because they are not exposed to it and often are not open to learning on their own. I was only able to get the message out to just so many doctors. In my opinion, the suppression of this vital information has led to the significant reduction of the quality and quantity of life for countless people who are suffering needlessly. This is not only wrong, but it is also dangerous, and in some cases even fatal.

As I said, going back to the early 1990s, I was noticing many more "off-label" benefits with Effexor XR (venlafaxine ER) than even the SSRIs, especially with regard to somatic and anxiety symptoms, such as reduction of headaches, neck, shoulder, and upper back pain and spasm; scattered joint pain such as fibromyalgia; IBS symptoms; pain and/or tension in whichever area of the body; etc.; and even ADD symptoms as well as energy and other benefits. I started treating the underlying disorder that was causing the symptoms rather than the usual treatment of symptomatic relief only. I did then and continue to prescribe SSRIs for the right patient, but usually they are the best second-line choices since more often than not SNRIs are the better first-line choices.

The SSRIs can also help somatic symptoms since if they improve depressive and anxiety symptoms, then this can also lead to improvement of physical symptoms, just not nearly as often. If one is not sure which class is better for an individual patient, then trying each separately can lead to the answer. Even if one is good, the other may be better. This is only discovered through the rational trial-and-error process.

Even though my patients and I were amazed at the difference they were seeing with Effexor XR (venlafaxine ER) as compared to the previous SSRIs, not everyone could tolerate it or needed it. Some had significant side effects that prohibited their use, and even if there were some positive benefits, they were not always worth the side effects. Even though some of them saw significant results, there were some that were still left unsatisfied. I knew with them that there was obviously something else going on, and I was determined to find out what it was.

In my first book, *Healing the Mind and Body,* I point out a few examples of standout results that I saw with Effexor XR (venlafaxine ER) that I hadn't seen previously. One was the woman with chronic vertigo for 30 years. She had been to many specialists and had been on many symptomatic medications that were totally resolved with the application of Effexor XR (venlafaxine ER). There was the woman with chronic recurring vaginal yeast infections that finally resolved after seeing gynecologists and infectious disease specialists hadn't helped, but rather she experienced excellent results regarding resolution of her infections after Effexor XR (venlafaxine ER) was taken. There was the man with chronic sciatica pain from chronic lower back pain. He even had been through a few surgeries at that point, which only provided short-term relief from the unrelenting pain. After Effexor XR (venlafaxine ER), his pain was managed with OTC anti-inflammatories and Tylenol, and he was able to stop the opiates that really weren't working that well anyway.

In some cases, the results were more dramatic than in other cases, but it was still remarkable to witness how much better certain people were getting. Patients who live with chronic pain, chronic stress, and emotional imbalance are relieved when the real underlying reason is successfully treated and when the need for treating the negative results from the underlying problems is not needed, or at least not as much. Instead of just "band-aiding" with medications that just cover up the symptoms, I found out that curing was even better and had more impact on people's lives. This makes for happy patients as well as happy doctors when we see the results and impact.

An Important Decision

By about the year 2000, the turn of the millennium, I had a difficult decision to make. I was witnessing firsthand such remarkable discoveries as I was treating more and more patients with this method of treating problems at their core. I was getting so busy treating psychosomatic disorders as well as other psychiatric disorders since I was getting so many referrals from patients, psychologists, and other doctors. I was getting too busy in a sense since I was also trying to continue seeing other primary care patients for many other regular issues. I realized that I was making a bigger difference in the quality of life of the patients I was treating for mind-body disorders than I was with other patients, who still got good results but not as impactful and exciting.

I was also recognizing and treating many different variants of bipolar disorder, which I will discuss further later in this book. I was learning augmentation strategies and polypharmaceutical techniques and strategies during the 1990s, which led to my methods regarding the rational approach that I employed. I was finding out that combining antidepressants with different mechanisms of action as well as combining antidepressants with mood stabilizers resulted in amazing results. I will also be discussing this further later in this book when I discuss the rational polypharmaceutical approach and the importance of achieving complete remission for all of our patients.

As I was saying, by the end of the previous and the beginning of a new millennium, I was getting so busy that I had to make the difficult decision to stop my regular primary care practice and focus all of my time on this subject. I still enjoyed doing primary care, but I found that it was not as interesting and impactful as what I was able to accomplish with the use of psychotropic medications. I found it challenging but also a lot of fun to work with these incredible tools in order to achieve results that I could not believe I was seeing. It was like solving complex living puzzles, and it was exciting to figure them out and complete them. As was the case with certain areas of medicine, I found this area to not be as routine, but rather more creative and interesting. I also felt that I was making a bigger difference. I saw that there were not a lot of doctors that really knew how to do this very well, so I saw that the need was so great that I decided to practice primary care psychiatry full-time.

This process of phasing out of regular primary care was difficult and painful at times, both for myself and for my patients, some of whom I had seen for many years. At that time, I was the owner of a group practice, with three or four other family doctors working with me. I was trying to transition a lot of patients to them so that I could open up my practice more to these specialty cases. I was still handling certain primary care problems, as I still occasionally do today, but I try to steer more away from that and focus on my field of expertise.

Even though I was continuing to treat some patients who had regular medical problems as well as psychosomatic problems, I only accepted new patients who had more psychiatric needs than other primary care patients. I had been working way too many hours (as my wife and kids can attest to), and I just couldn't do it anymore and had to use my time in the most effective way. I soon found that my practice was usually completely full, as I was doing what I love to do, trying to make the biggest difference that I could for the patients that were more challenging and fun to treat.

During the first decade of my practice, I was confused and shocked at times that more doctors didn't know about the miraculous results that I was seeing. There were a lot of "Oh my God" moments along the way when I saw certain things and was making breakthrough discoveries as to the specifics of how certain psychotropic medications affect certain patients in certain ways. I was seeing complex problems with certain patients that were literally being cured before my eyes with the simple use of these products. When I started seeing certain patterns in certain individuals, I was learning about the mind-body connection, which led to a lot of times that I thought, "If doing that means that," and then another "Oh my God" soon followed. I was seeing them then and have continued to make remarkable discoveries and breakthroughs the more I practiced and lectured. This then led me to start writing my first book in 2002, and I haven't stopped since. However, after 23 years of writing and six books, thankfully I am done.

I started to understand the subject in a unique way as a primary care doctor practicing full-time psychiatry, which I also refer to as mind-body medicine. I haven't met another doctor yet who has done that. I started seeing more and more of the stress-somatic link the more I practiced until I got it right.

I was amazed to be seeing complete resolution of many physical problems that I had not even really considered to be related to emotional problems. Once the cycle was broken by rebalancing neurochemicals within the nervous system, then this led to more complete results with proper treatment. As I said before, I understood by that point why other doctors were not picking up on this since, as I said, the lack of free speech because of the FDA and other governmental bodies means that most doctors never hear this information that could change their practice and improve the quality of life of their patients, which is sad.

This is a subject that is so important for not only primary care doctors and psychiatrists but for all other specialists too, since I can promise you that in some way stress affects the organ system that specialists are most interested in. We all see patients with mind-body disorders all the time, and it is important that they are understood and treated in the most compassionate and most ideal way by whichever physician, whether family physicians or internists, psychiatrists, or other specialists, as well as physician assistants (PAs) and nurse practitioners (NPs) who have the training to be able to understand and learn the importance of the mind-body connection and treating it in the most ideal preventative and holistic way with the use of psychotropic medications. My definition of holistic is helping the body to heal itself. That is exactly what psychotropic medications do. They simply balance neurochemicals only if they are out of balance in the first place, for reasons that the person has no control of. The result is holistic healing.

During the first decade of my practice I was voraciously reading, trying to figure this stuff out on my own since I really wasn't finding a lot of really practical and useful information about the subject. I pored through journals and read a few psychiatric textbooks, trying to keep up still with Family Practice CME (Continuing Medical Education) to keep my license up to date, and I spoke to certain doctors that I either lectured to, met at a conference somewhere, or saw at the hospital or at pharmaceutical dinners. I was trying to soak up as much information as I could since I was discovering so many interesting revelations as I was learning a lot by constantly practicing, and then I found out by a lot of trial-and-error that practice makes perfect.

I have spoken with a lot of psychiatrists, since usually I'm one of the only primary care doctors at speaker training conferences and other psychiatric meetings. I had also wondered during those years why the psychiatrists also didn't understand this, not just primary care doctors. I was fortunate to also speak to many primary care doctors, since they were usually the audience I was lecturing to, rather than psychiatrists.

I've seen some of the shortcomings of knowledge about this subject depending on one's specialty. Psychiatrists understand the mind very well but don't often understand its connection to the body. Primary care doctors understand a lot about the body but don't adequately appreciate the importance of the connection between the mind and the body, which comes out in emotional and physical ways. Specialists of whichever type typically focus on the organ system of their choice, though they need to understand the connection of whichever part of the body that they usually focus on and understand how that connects to the brain and how the physical symptoms tie in to emotions and mood. Since I did not lecture typically to psychiatrists, I have taken as much opportunity as possible to speak with the ones I see at pharmaceutical dinners or other places that psychiatrists hang out.

By about 2002, as I understood that I was not learning much by my research, I figured I should start writing down some ideas, which ended up being more than ideas. I started writing my first book, which I knew would be a long undertaking but one I felt compelled to share with others. I knew that what I was writing was completely unique, since if something like it were out there, I would probably have read it by then. I knew it would be a difficult undertaking, but I knew that I had to do it. I was compelled to share with others since it was such exciting news that I knew needed to be shared and understood by others. I wrote mostly weekends and some evenings at home between 2002 and 2007, while continuing a full-time clinical practice.[1] I wanted to share this phenomenon of treating the whole person at the same time: mind, body, and spirit.

We can learn to treat the physical problems and emotional problems in the same way since primary care doctors are supposed to be treating the whole person anyway. I also wanted to share this with mid-level practitioners such as PAs (physician assistants) and NP's (nurse practitioners). There are a significant number of them throughout the country, so it is very important that they understand how to treat these patients in the most optimal way. It is also very important for psychiatrists to learn how importantly the physical link ties into the emotional aspects of the body. I set out to share with all doctors, whether primary care, psychiatrists, or other specialists. I also wanted to share with psychologists the importance of understanding the role of psychotropic medications for their patients. I additionally wanted to reach out to other

1 I highly recommend a book that I read during this time (especially if you want to be a writer) by Stephen King called *On Writing*. One of his core messages is his advice to read every day and write every day. Simple advice but very profound. When I would get tired of writing and editing along the way I would take a break and read a book, but I was always back and forth between the two.

medical partners such as physical therapists, pharmacists, chiropractors, acupuncturists, and other ancillary providers. I also wanted to reach out to patients in order to give them something they could understand and then share with others, including their doctors. We all need to understand the critical nature of the subject, since we are all affected by it in one way or another.

I ended up writing more than I thought I would initially. Since after a few years I already had enough information for two books (about 80 pages), I focused on the first one for patients and the second more for doctors, but I had to focus on first things first. I finished the first book by 2007 and released it, took a much-needed break, and caught up on some reading, which really relaxes me. I then determined that the second one would be not only for doctors but also for patients who wanted to learn more than they learned in the first book. Between 2008 and 2014 the second book became too long at 800 pages, so I decided to separate it into two books; the second book more for patients and the third book more for doctors, but I also realized that doctors would need to read the first two in order to understand the third book. I also realized that patients would be able to understand at least parts of the third book and would find it interesting to see how and why doctors make the decisions that we do. I also envisioned that patients could educate their doctors by giving them the books so that their doctors could learn best how to help them. By 2014 I was 12 years into the writing process when I released my trilogy, weighing in at about 1,200 pages. I just had a lot to say, I guess.

That 12-year journey was difficult at times, as there was so much to do, but I kept my focus on the goal of completing what I had started. Since I was not seeing many doctors talk about this, I decided that I needed to say what needed to be said. I didn't hold back, and I wasn't politically correct (which I regard as a badge of honor) most of the time. I knew that what I needed to say wouldn't ever be approved by the FDA, so I didn't ask their permission. I wanted to be as honest as I could about the various presentations of neurochemical imbalances and that each individual has the rational hope of being cured if we do it correctly. Once we have hope, then everything changes and starts looking more positive with regard to the future. Once we get the mind and body working together, then we will see our patients getting completely better, resulting in the goal of mind-body harmony, which patients and doctors deserve to see after all their hard work and perseverance.

The Importance of Norepinephrine

Getting back on topic regarding what I was recognizing about how important norepinephrine was when I first experienced Effexor XR (venlafaxine ER) after the first three SSRIs, I was noticing that somatic symptoms were improving, anxiety symptoms were reducing, and overall mood was even better as compared to the SSRIs. I started to understand that norepinephrine was one of two neurochemicals that I target the most when I see patients who have somatic symptoms, an anxiety component, or just want overall better mood results. The other is GABA, which I will discuss in a bit.

The second SNRI released in 2004, a dozen years after I started practice, was a welcome addition that was a little different than Effexor XR (venlafaxine ER), but also very effective. After having so much experience with Effexor XR (venlafaxine ER) during the previous decade of my practice, I was ready for some competition that I could work with. The company Eli Lilly that launched Cymbalta (duloxetine) was smart since they studied its use with somatic symptoms such as fibromyalgia, neuropathy, and chronic pain disorders, and also found that it strengthened the bladder, resulting in less urinary leakage. It didn't surprise me because I knew why all that I was seeing with Cymbalta (duloxetine) was happening since I saw the same things with Effexor XR (venlafaxine ER) during the previous decade, including improvement of ADD symptoms, energy, and many other benefits. I was also excited that now I thought other doctors would pick up on this once they saw the results with Cymbalta (duloxetine).

Unfortunately, though, most doctors never really picked up on the importance of balancing norepinephrine and focused way too much time on serotonin. The fact that Cymbalta (duloxetine) got recognition as a treatment for fibromyalgia was huge, since this is such a mysterious medical problem to treat for most doctors. I figured that would mean that doctors would make the obvious leap towards recognizing the connection between the mind and body and thus see that it would be even easier to treat other somatic symptoms that are more chronic and low-grade, which also should be recognized and treated appropriately. I was recognizing how vastly important this subject was, and I felt desperate about the need to get this information out there. I was pleasantly surprised to see a somewhat enthusiastic audience when it was released, but it never really got the recognition that I hoped and prayed it would.

The problem is that since doctors did not by and large recognize the importance of balancing both serotonin and norepinephrine at the same time during the previous decade that the wonder drug Effexor XR (venlafaxine ER) had been out, then after the second one, the fact that there were now two medications out that helped both the mind and the body, doctors would recognize the importance of this subject and change their ways. Unfortunately, that was not the case.

Doctors initially got confused because in some cases Effexor XR (venlafaxine ER) is activating and increases energy. However, some people can feel a little jittery and nervous. Doctors mistook mild activating side effects that most people can adjust to for the perception that it increases anxiety and thus shouldn't be used for anxious patients. This was the exact opposite of the truth. In actuality I found it to be the best preventative antianxiety available, and usually more generally effective than SSRIs. I continued to be surprised as the years passed, surprised that other doctors were not picking up on the important preventative advantages that Effexor XR (venlafaxine ER) brought to the table. If they didn't really understand the first one, then it made sense that they wouldn't appreciate the second one.

I want to make it clear that I am by no means anti-SSRI, since I have prescribed them for many people for over more than three decades. However, the SSRIs were the first-line agents for far too many people. Most of them never got completely better. It is sad that there has been so much loss of opportunity for so many lives that otherwise have no hope. It is tragic that so many people do not have the opportunity to experience how their lives could be transformed for the better in easy and effective ways. The good news moving forward though, is that hope is alive for all who are in need.

As I said, I was more excited about the release of the second "classic" SNRI more than 10 years later. Effexor XR (venlafaxine ER) was and is a great medication, but it is not for everyone who needs an SNRI. Cymbalta (duloxetine) is less noradrenergic and more serotonergic than Effexor XR (venlafaxine ER), thus more balanced between these two neurochemicals. This can be helpful if Effexor XR (venlafaxine ER) is too activating, since this can be more calming. On the other hand, Effexor XR (venlafaxine ER) can help more with energy if that is needed and as long as the medication is tolerated. The bottom line, though, is that both are very good medications, and the proper choice really just depends on the needs of the individual.

I did a lot of "SNRI Taste Tests" during the first half of my practice when samples of both were available. I usually sent the patient home with both samples, and I usually started with the Effexor XR (venlafaxine ER) and then switched to Cymbalta (duloxetine) in order to figure out the details between the two. I found that about two-thirds or more of people chose Effexor XR (venlafaxine ER) over Cymbalta (duloxetine), but a third or so who chose Cymbalta (duloxetine) is still a lot of people. It was just so nice to have another option to work with.

Cymbalta (duloxetine) came out with doses of 20 mg, 30 mg, and 60 mg capsules. The recommended starting dose was 30 mg per day for one week and then 60 mg per day, though the company also said that starting with the most average dose of 60 mg was an alternative. The problem, though, is that this is like starting Effexor XR (venlafaxine ER) at 75 mg, which I would never do. I discovered that the 30 mg Cymbalta (duloxetine) was most equivalent to the 37.5 mg Effexor XR (venlafaxine ER), and in some even the 75 mg dose. I found the 60 mg Cymbalta (duloxetine) to be most equivalent to 75 mg of Effexor XR (venlafaxine ER), possibly up to 150 mg. For this reason, I have always started Cymbalta (duloxetine) at the 30 mg dose. I rarely have used the 20 mg dose, but that is reasonable if the patient is ultrasensitive and in need of a slower titration. The efficacy is seen within 2 to 4 days of a dose, as is the case with Effexor XR (venlafaxine ER) as well as the other SNRIs. 60 mg is the most common ending dose, with 30 mg the second most common, 90 mg the third most common, and 120 mg the least common dose. As is the case with Effexor XR (venlafaxine ER), Pristiq (desvenlafaxine), and Fetzima (levomilnacipran) (which I will discuss in a bit), the second lowest dose is also the most average one. It's important in this class to look closely at the first two doses since more likely than not one of them will be the final dose, though going higher can certainly benefit quite a few people.

Regarding Cymbalta (duloxetine), I have found it is more common with Effexor XR (venlafaxine ER) to see benefits at the higher dosage range than it is with Cymbalta (duloxetine), though I have many patients at higher levels of either of them. It just depends on the individual's need for balancing serotonin relative to norepinephrine, which is why one SNRI can be better than the other, which just depends on each individual's needs.

As I said earlier, what surprised me, though, is that even though the company that made Cymbalta (duloxetine) was able to market it for fibromyalgia since that was an "on-label" indication, it didn't make as significant of a difference as I thought it would. I figured that doctors would understand the message that even if a tough somatic problem like fibromyalgia is amenable to treatment, then they would understand that it would work for other somatic symptoms, right? I figured that they would understand that this was a class effect. Some doctors began to understand this more, but most doctors have been kept in the dark even to this day. It wasn't just a free speech issue. It was also a profound lack of understanding.

New and Improved

I was excited when Pristiq (desvenlafaxine) came out in 2008, and I was glad to be consulted by the company with a small group of doctors from around the country at a luxurious weekend at an out-of-state resort to get our opinions before it was formally launched. I was excited because it was being made by Wyeth, who originally made Effexor XR (venlafaxine ER) and Pristiq ER (desvenlafaxine succinate ER), which is the most active metabolite of Effexor XR (venlafaxine ER). I was told that this would be very effective, like its predecessor, but that it was even better tolerated and possibly had better efficacy. Since Effexor XR (venlafaxine ER) was already so good and I was getting very good results with Cymbalta (duloxetine) for many, it was certainly exciting to have a third SNRI available, since there were less than half as many SNRIs as SSRIs.

Pristiq (desvenlafaxine) has become the most prescribed medication over the last half of my practice, whereas Effexor XR (venlafaxine ER) was the most common medication I prescribed in the first half of my practice. Pristiq (desvenlafaxine) shares the characteristics of Effexor XR (venlafaxine ER) of being a bit more noradrenergic and a bit less serotonergic than Cymbalta (duloxetine), but it is a bit mellower and smoother, and sometimes a bit better tolerated than Effexor XR (venlafaxine ER), while the efficacy remains excellent. I did some Pristiq (desvenlafaxine)–Cymbalta (duloxetine) taste tests when Cymbalta (duloxetine) samples were available, so I was able to adequately compare the two to familiarize myself with the details of each product.

When Pristiq (desvenlafaxine) came out, there were again a couple of things that surprised me. One was that they didn't market it for somatic symptoms like fibromyalgia and other somatic disorders as Cymbalta (duloxetine) had, but they rather focused on major depressive disorder. It is certainly helpful for that, but that misses the whole point of what is different about balancing norepinephrine along with serotonin. If they would've studied it for headaches, IBS, fibromyalgia, other anxiety disorders, or other somatic symptoms, it would've gotten more indications than just the one.

Maybe they learned about the Cymbalta (duloxetine) launch; most doctors weren't understanding the difference between the two classes regarding somatic symptom reduction. It's also important to note and explain to patients that even though SNRIs are labeled as antidepressants, I much more commonly use them for anxiety disorders and/or somatic symptoms of whichever type, which are more common than depression, though depression may also be a factor since these diagnoses tend to travel together.

I tended to start with the Effexor XR (venlafaxine ER) or Pristiq (desvenlafaxine) and then switch to Cymbalta (duloxetine), since I wanted to try to avoid side effects in order to not scare the patient away. However, it is also reasonable to start with Cymbalta (duloxetine), since side effects of either are usually not severe and short-term, if any, and if the side effects are not tolerable, then the patient can switch to the other to see if it is better tolerated.

Effexor XR (venlafaxine ER) has the second-worst incidence of withdrawal side effects after Paxil (paroxetine), so it needs to be stopped gradually if it has been taken for a while. It may not be the best choice if the person has difficulty remembering to take a pill daily or otherwise misses frequently, such as forgetting to pack it when going out of town. Pristiq (desvenlafaxine) has a bit less of this potential withdrawal effect, but a bit more than Cymbalta (duloxetine). However, I have often found that if a person has difficulty getting off of an SNRI, then the person probably shouldn't be going off of it in the first place. I explain to them that we need to listen to what the body is telling us, since the body and mind are in control.

In my opinion the most interesting aspect of the Pristiq (desvenlafaxine) launch is that they came out with 50 and 100 mg tablets. It was clear to me soon after the release that 50 mg seemed to be too much to start with, based on quick efficacy but also side effects. I realized that starting at 50 mg was like starting Effexor XR (venlafaxine ER) at 75 mg or Cymbalta (duloxetine) at 60 mg, which I would never do. I kept a pill-splitting device on my desk and would cut two tablets in half and give those to the patient in a small folded piece of paper. I started them at 25 mg for four days and told them that if the results were excellent, then it was possible that 25 mg would be the ending dose. However, I then discovered that 50 mg is the average dose. The 25 mg dose is equivalent to the Effexor XR (venlafaxine ER) 37.5 mg and Cymbalta (duloxetine) 30 mg, with 50 mg being equivalent to Effexor XR (venlafaxine ER) 75 mg and possibly up to 150 mg or Cymbalta (duloxetine) 60 mg. Since the efficacy of an SNRI is seen within 2 to 4 days of a dose, quick decisions can be made with regard to finding the optimal dose. I was thankful that when

Pristiq (desvenlafaxine) came out with the generic, they released a 25 mg tablet so that I could put away the pill-splitter.

What I have shared are some of the details regarding the first three SNRIs, but the actual response is so individualized that it is difficult to generalize which one is the best for each individual patient. Overall, in my experience, though, Pristiq (desvenlafaxine) is the best of the three, but only by a little bit. What surprised me most about the Pristiq (desvenlafaxine) launch was that they did not study it or market it for somatic symptom reduction, which I feel was a missed opportunity. Maybe they realized that it really didn't make that much of a difference since most doctors did not understand the message with Cymbalta (duloxetine), so why bother? They probably realized that the FDA would not allow any free speech about "off-label" content. I wonder, though, if they would have studied it for somatic symptoms, then maybe the truth would have been discovered? We will never know. However, if they would have marketed it as it should have by mentioning somatic symptom reduction, anxiety improvement, and overall better efficacy for depression, then possibly the reasons why dual-action agents are better than single-action agents would have been realized more, but then again, maybe not.

The Fourth and Final "Classic" SNRI?

The fourth and final SNRI that came out in 2013 is Fetzima (levomilnacipran), and its key characteristic is that it has a 2 to 1 ratio of balancing norepinephrine more than serotonin; thus, I consider it an NSRI. This can be good for those patients who have more somatic and higher anxiety symptoms and can tolerate one of the other three in this class. The problem, though, is that it may be too noradrenergic, thus leading to side effects such as activation, dry mouth, constipation, urinary retention, and nausea. However, I don't mean to overstate the side effects because the truth is that overall all of the medications in this class are very good and usually well-tolerated, and if not, then another one in this class can be chosen as appropriate, which is the case when norepinephrine is significantly imbalanced in the individual. If noradrenergic side effects, however, are significant, then this likely means that an SNRI that is less noradrenergic or an SSRI may be the better choice.

The message when Fetzima (levomilnacipran) was launched also unfortunately focused on the indication for major depressive disorder, with not enough discussion of fibromyalgia or other somatic symptoms. I was glad to see that it came in four doses of 20 mg, 40 mg, 80 mg, and 120 mg capsules. This showed the recognition that lower, midrange, and higher doses are all needed. When it was first launched, the recommended titration was to start with 20 mg for two days and then 40 mg per day, which is how the initial sample pack came out. They fell into the same trap of trying to titrate it quickly in order to get the quickest efficacy in order to help market this benefit, however, the message soon shifted when it was realized that titration was too fast.

They then came out with one-week samples of only 20 mg, with separate one-week samples of 40 mg and the two higher doses. Since this medication has double the balancing of norepinephrine compared to serotonin, it is a bit more likely that 20 mg would be the ideal dose more often than the lower dose of the others. However, the most common ending dose appears to be 40 mg, with the second most common dose 20 mg, with 80 mg the third most common dose and 120 mg the least common dose. This is the exact same message as the other three: the fact that lower is often better than higher when it comes to this class.

The most recent SNRI taste test was when samples of both Pristiq (desvenlafaxine) and Fetzima (levomilnacipran) were available. I soon discovered that Pristiq (desvenlafaxine) 25 mg was equivalent to Fetzima (levomilnacipran) 20 mg, Pristiq (desvenlafaxine) 50 mg was equivalent to Fetzima (levomilnacipran) 40 mg, and Pristiq (desvenlafaxine) 100 mg was equivalent to the Fetzima (levomilnacipran) 80 mg to 120 mg range. If anxiety and somatic symptoms are still present with Pristiq (desvenlafaxine), sometimes this would improve when switching to Fetzima (levomilnacipran) since it is more noradrenergic. This can be a good move as long as the Fetzima (levomilnacipran) is tolerated.

Even if another "classic" SNRI doesn't come out, the four that we already have available provide more than adequate choices that are usually good enough to do the job well, which is important because SNRIs are the best first-line choice that we have available for the majority of people that we see.

* * * * *

During the first half of my practice in the 1990s and early 2000s, I was told by the representative that I was the top prescriber of Effexor XR (venlafaxine ER), and over the last half of my practice, I am also now the top prescriber of Pristiq (desvenlafaxine). I'm not surprised about this since I have learned to use these medications in so many different ways. They have been my first-line agents since the beginning of my practice, since I start with the best in order to find the ideal first agent before augmenting from there. It's really best to build upon a good foundation. In one sense, though, I'm saddened that I prescribe them so much more than others because this just means that not enough doctors understand the importance of mind-body balancing.

The reason I started using Pristiq (desvenlafaxine) more was because samples were available when they stopped giving me Effexor XR (venlafaxine ER) samples. It is very useful to be able to give samples of the medication at the office. This can improve compliance by being able to avoid the pharmacy at the beginning, since some people may just not go, or some may be given a handout by the pharmacy that scares them into not taking it. Once I show patients the results, then they are less likely to be swayed by reading imbalanced and harmful information that the FDA forces the company to say.

If the patient goes to the pharmacy or tries to look up a medication online, I warn them ahead of time to be cautious about what they read, since I can give them much more useful and practical information than they'll receive by reading mostly negative information. I warn patients that reading too much is like getting medical advice from an attorney instead of a doctor, which I don't recommend.

Other Noradrenergic Options

We also have other medication choices that focus on blocking the reuptake of norepinephrine, thus encouraging its forward flow throughout the nervous system, though I tend to use them less than the "classic" SNRIs. Remeron (mirtazapine) is a good medication that balances norepinephrine as well as serotonin but also has a strong effect on histamine, which can lead to side effects such as fatigue and weight gain. It can be a very good choice to treat insomnia.

Wellbutrin (bupropion) is an nDRI, which definitely focuses more on dopamine but also has a lesser norepinephrine effect, which is still significant, making it the most ideal augmenting medication that I have worked with over the years.

Tricyclic antidepressants are what I refer to as the "old-school" SNRIs, since they were efficacious partly due to the dual action of balancing serotonin and norepinephrine at the same time. The problem with the tricyclics was and is overall tolerance, which can make them difficult to work with, especially at higher and more efficacious doses. The most common side effects are nausea, sweating, constipation, urinary retention, dry mouth, fatigue, cognitive side effects, and a potential suicide risk if one overdoses and other problems.

Where they tend to be most useful is when adding low doses of the tricyclics with SSRIs in order to have an augmenting effect on sleep, pain, and anxiety reduction. However, even at low doses they can be problematic, which limits their use. I utilize them on occasion, but rarely since I have found other better options, especially the "classic" SNRIs that improve both somatic and emotional symptoms. We can thus kill two birds with one stone since with one medication it is usually even better than the dual combination of an SSRI with a tricyclic antidepressant, with better efficacy, compliance, and fewer side effects. The positive effects are the same, such as preventative reduction of pain and anxiety, along with benefits for sleep, energy, and overall mood. An SNRI is a win-win medication.

Strattera (atomoxetine) is an NRI (norepinephrine reuptake inhibitor), with a slight reuptake inhibition of dopamine. It is a decent medication, especially if a stimulant is not tolerated or there is concern about addiction, but it is overall not as efficacious as the stimulants are. It's a decent first-line choice but may be a better option than a stimulant if a stimulant is not tolerated or if there is a contraindication such as certain cardiac issues. It may be a good augmenting agent with the stimulants Wellbutrin XL and others. Since it balances norepinephrine, it may reduce somatic symptoms and anxiety symptoms.

Qelbree (viloxazine) is the second non-stimulant NRI, and also has a lesser effect on dopamine, as is the case with Strattera (atomoxetine), but this product also has an agonist boosting effect on serotonin, unlike Strattera (atomoxetine). At the time of this writing, I haven't had much experience with it yet since it recently came out. As is the case with Strattera (atomoxetine), I would consider it as first-line if stimulants are not tolerated, if addiction is a concern, or if there are any medical contraindications when it comes to taking a stimulant.

Stimulants, though, are the "gold standard" treatment of ADD/ADHD, and it is difficult to beat their efficacy. They also, in my opinion, decrease the risk of addiction to not only stimulants but also other addictive substances. This leads to being evaluated on a case-by-case basis, since addiction to prescription stimulants can occur. If the patient truly has ADD/ADHD, then the risk of addiction is minimal. If the person does not have this diagnosis, however, then the risk of addiction is higher, however that person is more likely to desire the street versions and not the prescription ones. They are cheaper and easier to obtain. It doesn't take a doctor visit or a prescription to get methamphetamines, and addicts tend to prefer it.

If the person truly has ADD/ADHD, stimulants should actually be calming (unless the dose is too high) and not activating/stimulating and usually reduce anxiety and depression and improve overall mood in general. Stimulants focus on dopamine and norepinephrine by stimulating them to move forward and even slightly attach to these receptor sites and help to block the abnormal reuptake of these neurochemicals, though antidepressants do an even better job of doing that. This is why I often add antidepressants to stimulants for a boosting effect. This is particularly the case with Wellbutrin XL, but also potentially with an SNRI or one of the two NRIs.

When one feels the boost of mood and reduction of anxiety, then the risk of addiction is minimized. Psychotropic medications in general actually calm the brain as well as activate it when either is needed. They are truly the best preventative anti-addiction medications currently available, which are not habit-forming and are extremely safe and effective.

The Journey Forward

In my third book of the *Healing the Mind and Body* trilogy series, I categorize and discuss all of the antidepressants. I have a separate section for the SNRIs in which I discussed each medication in great detail, as well as discussing the different taste tests that are available to try. I also discuss SNRIs frequently in my first two books, since they were the first cornerstone of my practice. Instead of going into too many details, as is the case with the second chapter of my third book, in this book I wanted to discuss this class in more generalized and practical terms. The reason that I am telling my story from the beginning is so that you can see how and why I learned what I did each step of the way, which has been an incredible journey of discovery that has been exciting to travel.

As I have already said, the lack of recognition by the so-called "experts" who believe that SSRIs are the best first-line agents for the majority of patients is just plain wrong. Treating depression and anxiety along with somatic symptoms is one of the core messages of all of my books, and I discovered this over 30 years ago. When I saw with my own eyes the importance of balancing norepinephrine in addition to serotonin by witnessing the results firsthand, I was hooked.

This is especially true when it comes to unipolar disorder. However, we can also use them for the treatment of anxiety disorders, ADD/ADHD and bipolar disorder, since other diagnoses often accompany depression, in actuality, most of the time.

Once I started recognizing the power of a dual-action medication that balances serotonin and norepinephrine, then I opened up to other augmentation strategies. I started seeing how amazing the results were and how powerful the possibilities were when it comes to making the best first-line choice as well as choosing an augmenting agent, which leads to the best results both emotionally and physically. The rational polypharmaceutical approach leads to truly impressive results with surprising ease.

An SNRI is the most likely psychotropic medication to achieve remission or at least a response with a solo agent. It's important to make sure that we make the best first selection since the overall results will be better if we are building on a solid foundation before we then turn our attention to choosing the best augmenting agent. The remission rate is about 40 to 45% when it comes to efficacy in the treatment of unipolar disorder, with SSRIs following at 30 to 35%. However, this also means that more than half of patients need the addition of a second medication in order to achieve the goal of complete and full remission, which just happens to be the goal for every patient that we see.

Another misconception is that SNRIs should not be used if the patient has bipolar disorder, but I have found that usually is not the case. It really depends on the degree of the problem. Since the majority of bipolar disorder is spent in depression and not in mania or even hypomania, it makes sense to use whichever antidepressant we would use with unipolar disorder, which likely means an SNRI first-line. It's more likely, though, in many cases of bipolar disorder—more often than in unipolar disorder—that an SSRI and/or Wellbutrin XL are more attractive choices. It depends on the level of somatic symptoms as well as the anxiety component. It is important though, to understand that it really depends on the severity of the bipolar condition. In other words, with Bipolar I Disorder or Schizoaffective Disorder, we need to proceed with caution when it comes to antidepressants in general and rather focus on mood stabilization first and then antidepressants at the right time. This is also the case, though less so with Bipolar II Disorder. In some patients with Bipolar I an antidepressant is not even needed, though that is less common than the usual case. These choices really just depend on the individuality of that person.

The reality is that getting the antidepressant right is critical if one wants to achieve true remission. If that is the case, then the addition of an SNRI may work well, but if there is concern that it may be too "activating," then this may necessitate increasing one or more of the mood stabilizers to help to balance things out. If any antidepressant destabilizes the patient, then it can always be stopped, or the dose can be lowered.

It's important to try to find a balance between the mind and body, and if an imbalance of norepinephrine is a significant factor, then it is important to address the physical and emotional connection by balancing norepinephrine if needed and then seeing which augmentation strategy is best, with the goal of full remission always in mind.

GABA-DABA-DOO

The final chapter I will discuss in this section concerns my discovery that, even when norepinephrine and serotonin (and even dopamine) were previously balanced, many patients still had residual symptoms related to somatic symptoms, anxiety symptoms, underlying depression, and other negative mood states. I already understood dopamine when I was augmenting with Wellbutrin XL or with a dopamine antagonist, with both often combined together in order to form an exciting medication combination, balancing dopamine 24/7. I discovered that this was very important with regard to quality-of-life symptoms, resolution of mania and hypomania, improvement of depressive symptoms, and other problems related to mood disorders such as energy, sleep, focus, concentration, executive functioning, and other potential benefits.

However, when I discovered the role of GABA (gamma-aminobutyric acid), I realized that its imbalance was the missing piece of the puzzle when it comes to the resolution of somatic symptoms, anxiety-related symptoms, and residual depression, as well as hypomania and/or mania. I first started understanding the GABA/glutamate agents in the early 1990s, about the same time when I was beginning to understand the importance of Effexor XR (venlafaxine ER).

GABA is the main inhibitory neurochemical, so improving the forward flow of GABA has a calming effect on the nervous system. Glutamate is the main excitatory neurochemical, so suppressing and reducing the flow also leads to calming of the nervous system. Boosting glutamate and/or reducing the flow of GABA leads to an activating and energized state. Auvelity (Dextromethorphan/Bupropion SR) is a new and exciting antidepressant with the unique action of boosting glutamate with dextromethorphan, with the other half being Wellbutrin SR, which boosts mostly dopamine but also norepinephrine. It is also a sigma-1 receptor agonist, which appears to have a slight boosting effect on serotonin and norepinephrine. I typically augment first with Wellbutrin XL, but if this does not work adequately, meaning it works but then "poops out," then this is an excellent choice. It is a very powerful and stimulating agent, which I reserve for treatment-resistant depression, which is not uncommon.

My earliest experience with a GABA agent was with gabapentin/neurontin, and I understood quite well that it helped with pain as well as with anxiety, but I was also seeing that it was a decent, mild mood stabilizer at the same time, which I found to be quite convenient and helpful. It is frequently used by neurologists for many different reasons, and it is also popular with pain specialists, as well as primary care doctors and psychiatrists. It was good for patients who have been overdependent on benzodiazepines and sleeping pills, for difficult and chronic pain conditions, neurological symptoms such as neuropathy and others, as well as other benefits that came with the reduction of anxiety and other mood-related benefits. It had the flexibility of being able to work at low doses and high doses, depending on the needs of the individual. Some have to deal with fatigue, cognitive side effects, and weight gain, though overall it is well-tolerated if it is chosen for the right individual. As good as it initially was, though, I ended up discovering an even better choice.

Topamax (topiramate) was an early discovery that came out in the mid-1990s, and I figured out quickly the "off-label" benefit of migraine headache prevention. The FDA eventually recognized this indication in 2004, and it was then considered on-label. I also discovered, though, that not only did it help prevent migraine headaches, but this also helped not only to prevent migraine headaches but also with tension/muscular headaches, neck, shoulder, and upper back pain, lower back pain, fibromyalgia, IBS, or whichever residual somatic symptoms are not resolved by just balancing norepinephrine.

When it comes to somatic and/or anxiety symptoms, I usually think of norepinephrine first, but GABA comes in at a close second. Serotonin and dopamine may also play a role with somatic and mood symptoms. However, the SNRI-GABAergic combination is one of the original "Dynamic Duos." I also discovered that this combination helped with anxiety symptoms and the reduction of depressive symptoms, as well as the resolution of somatic symptoms, all at the same time. This was an exciting discovery of tremendous importance.

The advantage Topamax (topiramate) has over most of the other GABA agents is that it reduces weight by reducing the desire for sugars, carbohydrates, and sodas. It can also reduce the cravings for alcohol and other illicit drugs. The reduction of weight is often helpful with these patients since they may be on medications that tend towards weight gain. Adding Topamax (topiramate) can thus help mitigate some of the side effects.

Its biggest problem is cognitive side effects and possibly fatigue, though these may be balanced by other medications such as Wellbutrin, stimulants, Provigil (modafinil), Nuvigil (armodafinil), Sunosi (solriamfetol), Deplin (L-methylfolate), and others. The cognitive effects may just be dose-related, so it depends if efficacy is achieved prior to the onset of this or other side effects. Though it's certainly not for everybody, this medication is a godsend, as it is unique in its action and unlike any other augmentation strategy.

I have also used Depakote frequently over the years, which is a more potent GABA/glutamate agent and one of the "classic" mood stabilizers (along with lithium carbonate), as well as Trileptal (oxcarbazepine), Tegretol (carbamazepine), Keppra (levetiracetam), Lamictal (lamotrigine) and others. Depakote is known for migraine headache prevention, though it is a bit more heavy-handed than Topamax (topiramate) and has weight gain instead of weight loss as a potential side effect, so it would be reserved for more severe cases. Trileptal (oxcarbazepine) is also a very good mood stabilizer and is nice to have as an augmenting agent. Lamictal (lamotrigine) is well-known for its effectiveness in stabilizing mood and treating bipolar depression. As an invaluable and very unique medication, I have often added it to a regimen to bring patients with bipolar spectrum disorders into remission by resolving cyclical depression. I continue to augment with whatever is needed in order to optimally balance both the mind and body at the same time in order to achieve the ultimate goal of mind-body harmony.

SECRET #2

Recognizing the Full Range of Bipolar Disorder, From the Obvious to the More Subtle Variations of Bipolar Spectrum Disorder

SECRET #2

Recognizing the Full Range of Bipolar Disorder, From the Obvious to the More Subtle Variations of Bipolar Spectrum Disorder

In order to understand this issue, I need to take you back to the early 1990s when I started practice. As I previously said, I was already understanding the importance of the dual action of serotonin and norepinephrine with regard to all the different mind-body presentations. I was prescribing Effexor XR (venlafaxine ER) like it was going out of style. I was seeing the amazing presentations and results after treatment, and this changed everything. I want to make it clear, though, that I am by no means anti-SSRI. I have a lot of people that I have prescribed them to with good results, though I consider them second-line medications more often than not.

I was also beginning to understand the role of GABA, with early experience prescribing Topamax (topiramate), Gabapentin, Depakote, and others. I was understanding unipolar disorder very well thanks to Effexor XR (venlafaxine ER) as well as combining it with Wellbutrin XL and other exciting augmenting agents that we have to work with.

What I was seeing, though, was that some of the patients were more difficult to treat and took longer to get better or just didn't completely get better. They had mood fluctuations, which present with mood swings and instability. Antidepressants alone didn't seem to completely do the job. Some got worse with antidepressants, or antidepressants only gave incomplete results that were not yet satisfying. Some would get better for a while, and then a few months later "poop-out," (I know it's a very technical term and also quite descriptive). The medications just stopped working for some strange reason.

There are patients that need more "band-aid" medications such as tranquilizers (benzodiazepines), sleeping pills, pain pills, or any other products that treat symptoms by covering them up rather than getting to the underlying core of the problem. They also tended to require higher doses for the more symptomatic patients, whereas unipolar patients often require lower doses only, and even often PRN (as needed) and not daily. Bipolar patients often have more "loaded" family histories, often on both sides, whereas unipolar patients may have a significant history only on one side. They also tend to have more problems that are more difficult to resolve than patients with strictly unipolar disorder, which presents more simply and is more easily treated. There is a fine line between unipolar disorder and bipolar disorder, so we need to appreciate the subtleties and understand how to treat each individual in the most complete way. The difference between unipolar and bipolar can be very subtle, and it can be difficult to recognize the separation between the two because they coexist in many people.

My first exposure to bipolar disorder was in the late 1980s to early 1990s, which was during my years of training as well as early private practice. I had a special interest and curiosity regarding the treatment of mood disorders. The word got out, and I was getting a lot of referrals from nutritionists, psychologists, and doctors to treat eating disorders such as anorexia nervosa and bulimia nervosa. I got a lot of early experience treating these and other more complex and difficult-to-treat patients. The more I learned about them, the easier it was to treat other more common patients with easier-to-treat presentations. Treating unipolar disorder was certainly exciting, and I found that it was also simpler to treat.

Patients with Bipolar Disorder I found were more complex and a bit more difficult to treat, which was interesting since it was more challenging but also fun to see such dramatic results, even more so than some of the bipolar patients. We can even make a bigger difference in their lives. Even the "Dynamic Duo" (an SNRI-Wellbutrin XL combination) wasn't working adequately. I noticed that antidepressants only got them so far but did not get them to the finish line of full and complete remission.

Early on I was discovering that Risperdal (risperidone) was getting many of these complicated patients into remission. I didn't really know how to label what I was seeing or treating at that point, but I just went with my gut and developed a feel for it. They didn't really present with typical bipolar features, or what I thought bipolar disorder meant at that time, so I did not really think of it in those terms but rather that it was an augmenting tool that was helping patients who were already taking antidepressants and were not getting completely better. It was obviously stabilizing their moods as well as improving their depressive symptoms at the same time. I noticed that it was helping both ends of the spectrum, which was interesting and exciting.

Risperdal (risperidone) came out in 1994, which was two years after my clinical practice started, and was the first "atypical" antipsychotic, meaning that it not only works as a dopamine antagonist but also works as a serotonin antagonist at the same time. It was originally indicated for schizophrenia before it later became indicated for bipolar disorder. It was better tolerated overall than its predecessors, with sometimes even better mood results. It also had a significantly reduced chance of extrapyramidal symptoms, the worst being tardive dyskinesia. The reality, though, is that I have not seen one case of TD since Risperdal (risperidone) came out, as is the case also with all of the others that have come out since then. We may see akathisia and other lesser extrapyramidal symptoms, though these issues are easier to resolve by lowering the dose or stopping it.

I was noticing, though, that Risperdal (risperidone) had some significant side effects for some, including oversedation, hyperprolactinemia (with potential milk discharge from the breasts and potential breast enlargement in women and men, though this is not a common side effect), weight gain, and others. However, for most patients the good far outweighs the bad.

During the early to mid 1990s I was getting so much experience with Risperdal (risperidone) that the company sent me to a speaker training conference and trained me to lecture to primary care doctors. I welcomed the opportunity, since I was so excited to share with them what I had already seen happening with its use. I spoke with them about bipolar disorder, but that condition really didn't define the majority of the symptoms I was seeing with my patients. I was often not seeing mania as much as hypomania, which can easily be misdiagnosed as unipolar anxiety if one doesn't notice the subtleties. However, depression was the obvious dominant symptom for most people, along with symptoms of anxiety and other stress-related somatic symptoms. The treatment for mania was certainly impressive, since it improved this more as the dose was increased and was usually fairly well-tolerated. What was more impressive, though, was that the depressive symptoms were also responding.

Back then I could speak about "off-label" benefits without worrying about the consequences. I shared what I saw was really happening, which most of the time was different than the indication it originally was meant for. They seemed receptive to the message, and I had really hoped that it would change their habits. The psychiatrists seemed to understand it more than the family physicians, but even the psychiatrists did not seem to have a full appreciation of the importance of the subject of emotional and physical improvements at the same time, and I noticed that they did not always appreciate that depression seemed to be the most common symptom that was resolved with Risperdal (risperidone).

I was seeing such dramatic results with my patients that I continued to practice combining mood stabilizers and antidepressants until I started to understand how vast and important the bipolar spectrum really was. I was noticing how commonly this occurs in a primary care practice, probably even more so than in the office of the psychiatrist, since the presentations more often include the body and not just the brain. Psychiatrists often see somatic symptoms but don't always necessarily understand them and know what to do about them.

As I said, I didn't really know what I was treating back then, so I just followed my gut instincts and developed a feel for what I was doing. I knew that by witnessing the results firsthand and seeing what an impact was made, I knew that this method and protocol were working better than any other method that I had previously studied in the literature. What I discovered was that there was a lot more going on between unipolar and bipolar disorders than was evident at the surface, so I started to dig deeper and explore.

A BIG Breakthrough

A big breakthrough happened in 1997 when I was invited to a speaker training meeting in Chicago about bipolar disorder, focusing on speaking to primary care doctors about the subject. I thought I knew what bipolar disorder was when I went to that conference, but I soon found out that I only understood part of the story. I discovered that it was way more common than I had originally thought.

I've been to several weekend speaker training conferences, and most of them were tolerable and were meant to train us to use the slide deck and practice our presentations. There usually wasn't a lot of new or interesting cutting-edge information, so I enjoyed many relaxing weekends in my own hotel room in order to catch up on some reading while enjoying good food and drink and catching up on sleep.

The conference in Chicago regarding speaking to primary care physicians about using Zyprexa (olanzapine) for bipolar disorder was definitely way different than the norm. From the opening speaker, my interest was piqued when I was listening to what he was saying. I started looking for paper since

I wasn't prepared to take notes, and then I wrote as quickly as I could as I tried to keep up with what I was hearing.

By the time the second and third speakers came on, I was hooked, since this information was definitely new and different, and I realized how impactful it really was. I ended up writing a lot of material that weekend, and on the plane ride home I organized all my notes, which became the basis of the bipolar chapter in my first book, "The Ups and Downs of Bipolar Disorder," as well as writings on the subject in all six books.

That weekend I was able to converse with a lot of doctors and compare notes. I shared my ideas about what I was seeing, and I listened intently to other doctors as they shared their experiences. I remember being unsatisfied and frustrated since I couldn't find any other doctors who could understand what I was sharing with them about my experiences and what I was seeing, which was that many of the patients we thought had unipolar disorder actually had certain variations of bipolar disorder instead. This conference was certainly a breakthrough for me of far-reaching implications.

During that weekend in Chicago there were a lot of "Oh my God" moments, and these continued as I put into practice what I had learned as I was witnessing miracle after miracle before my eyes. Even the most difficult cases got better. I started really appreciating the augmenting power that atypical antipsychotics provide. They are powerful tools that we can employ when we try to get patients to full remission.

Since it is a mood stabilizer, it works on both ends of the spectrum by controlling the mania and hypomania as well as the depression and other symptoms in between. I started using Zyprexa (olanzapine) over and over again and was amazed at the positive results I saw in virtually all of the patients we called into the office after I came back from that weekend.

It worked better than Risperdal (risperidone) in some patients and was very well-tolerated and gentle. It was mildly sedating, so it would normally be dosed in the evening, as it would help with sleep, anxiety, and mood, whether high or low. It was more well-rounded than Risperdal (Risperidone) since it has action at multiple receptor sites.

The big problem, though, that I discovered over time was that Zyprexa (olanzapine) caused too much weight gain for a lot of people, which was unfortunate because that was the only real fault of the medication. It is still an excellent medication for certain patients, such as those who are very sensitive to medications and those who may benefit from an increased appetite and increased weight.

The next big moment came when Seroquel (quetiapine) and Seroquel XR (Quetiapine ER) came out in 1997. I was excited to have a third modern atypical to work with, since I discovered that the first two weren't always the answer. The most noticeable aspect of this product was how good it was for people who have insomnia, whether mild, moderate, or severe, and whether acute or chronic. There's no more effective psychotropic medication when it comes to sleep quality in my experience.

Seroquel (quetiapine) and Seroquel XR (quetiapine ER) were effective for mania, especially at high doses, though they only typically require lower doses in order to get the sleep benefit, and raising the dose too high can lead to lingering sedation the next day. One handy trick though in this situation is to add Wellbutrin XL in the morning, which boosts dopamine, which results in improved daytime energy. Seroquel (quetiapine) and Seroquel XR (quetiapine ER) offered a wide range of dosing, from low to medium to high, and the ideal dose for the individual is figured out along the way. We need to optimize benefits while minimizing side effects, with the ending dose really up to the body. I often use low-dose Seroquel (quetiapine) or Seroquel XR (quetiapine ER) to help with sleep quality because it is extremely effective for that purpose. Often though that is not enough to treat the underlying bipolar disorder. I often combine two atypical antipsychotic medications together in order to maximize the benefits of both while avoiding the side effects of increasing either of them too high. A common example is using Seroquel for its sleep benefit, and in case we cannot get the dose high enough to get mood stabilization, then I would add a second. There are other examples also.

I enjoyed getting away to the speaker training conferences that I attended to prepare for speaking with primary care doctors about this product. I asked a lot of questions and challenged the speakers during the smaller group sessions to give me better information as to why they weren't talking about what I had been seeing in clinical practice. I also wondered why they were marketing it at a higher dose with an aggressive dosing strategy rather than the low and slow approach that I preferred.

I had also noticed that it helped with depression and anxiety symptoms, since it's a true mood stabilizer. It is also histaminergic, which contributes to fatigue. Seroquel (quetiapine) and Seroquel XR (quetiapine ER) ended up being too sedating for some, which meant that the dose could not get to the therapeutic level needed due to the somnolence.

Seroquel XR (quetiapine ER) came out in 2007, but it really wasn't a big deal since the medication is no different and just has a time-released coating, which slowed down the sedation and didn't have the "punch" regarding the onset of sleep as the first version, Seroquel IR (instant release), had.

Seroquel (quetiapine) was and is an excellent medication, one that I have prescribed about the most in my career. However, due to the weakness of excessive drowsiness for some, as well as some weight gain for certain patients (as was the case with Risperdal (risperidone) and Zyprexa (olanzapine), with Zyprexa (olanzapine) being the top offender regarding weight gain). I was looking forward to having other upcoming choices. Even though these first three modern atypical agents were overall excellent choices for many, I was really excited when the next one came out.

New and Exciting

The next groundbreaking product that then came out was Abilify (Aripiprazole) in 2002, which ended up being a huge hit. It was different than the first three in that it was not usually too sedating and was often more energizing than the others. This is because it is not only a dopamine D2 antagonist as well as a serotonin antagonist like all the others but also a dopamine and serotonin partial agonist, meaning that they don't always go backwards but also move somewhat in a forward direction, as is the case with some of the more modern atypical antipsychotics that I will discuss in a bit.

Since fatigue is one of the biggest side effect problems with this class in general, it was nice when a less sedating option came out. It was calming and mildly sedating for some, and in that case, I would dose it in the evening. In others it was more energizing/activating, so in their cases they took it in the morning. It usually doesn't matter when it's taken, and if that's the case, the person can take it when it's most convenient.

Some patients had problems with akathisia, but this is usually dose-related. It does have a higher akathisia rate than many of the other atypicals, but it's usually not a problem.

It can be too activating and energizing in some, which may present as anxiety. In some it can be sedating, so it's difficult to tell until we try it on an individual and see what happens. Initially it was touted as having a low risk of weight gain, but I soon discovered that wasn't always the case and that some people had significant weight gain, which, besides akathisia and being overly sedating is the other biggest problem with this class of medications in general.

As is always the case, the company initially touted a too-quick and too-high dosage message, and we soon discovered these recommendations were too aggressive and really only spoke to one aspect of bipolar disorder, which is mania (with psychotic presentations at times), as well as schizophrenia.

As I learned with the first three atypicals, the dosing needs to be slowed down to account for patients with lower-grade bipolar disorder, not just higher-grade. I found that lower doses were the best for many patients with lesser presentations, where depression is way more common than mania or hypomania.

As was the case with the previous atypicals, this also had a positive mood benefit with regard to depression and anxiety disorders. When the dose is pushed higher, it also helps more with controlling not only mania and hypomania but also the more severe forms of depressive symptoms. This is the case with all of the mood stabilizers, since they focus on both ends of the spectrum.

Around the same time that Abilify (aripiprazole) came out, Geodon (ziprasidone) was also introduced. I had some good experiences with it, but it is a bit more difficult to work with, and there was concern about the potential for Q-T prolongation and the potential need to monitor EKGs. However, I discovered that this risk was way overblown and that practically one does not need to do so. An advantage with this product was that it was one of the least likely to cause weight gain, which is a distinct advantage since most atypicals do the opposite. It is not only an antagonist at dopamine D2 but also norepinephrine and is also an antagonist at serotonin 5HT2A and 5HT1D, with agonist effects at 5HT1A. As is the case with Abilify (Aripiprazole), the agonist effect is probably why it is not usually sedating. I have had so much experience with the other atypicals and have less experience with this one, though it is still a very good option.

Invega (paliperidone) came out in 2006 by the makers of Risperdal (risperidone), and to create Invega (paliperidone), they tweaked Risperdal (risperidone) to make it better by lowering the risk of hyperprolactinemia, sedation, and weight gain. It's a very good product, though I have tended to prescribe others in this class more. There are just so many good choices.

Saphris (asenapine) then came out, which was sedating, but less so than Seroquel (quetiapine), Seroquel XR (quetiapine ER), and some of the others. It had the biggest variety of receptor site activity among the atypical class. It also had the advantage of less potential for weight gain than some of the others besides Geodon (ziprasidone). It dissolves under the tongue, so this was a feature that some patients didn't care for, since the taste isn't great, though for most who take it, this is not a big issue.

Fanapt (iloperidone) came out around that time, but I discovered that it was a very potent antipsychotic and more appropriate for severe cases, so I really didn't get much experience prescribing it since the indication was schizophrenia. However, more recently it has been released for the indication of Bipolar I Disorder, and since then I have found it to be a good medication, also with a low potential for weight gain. The company does what all of them do, by recommending a quick titration by starting it twice a day and increasing it fairly quickly. Instead, I slow down the titration by half and dose it only in the evening to avoid daytime side effects such as short-term dizziness at the beginning that the person usually adjusts to quickly. The ending dose also may be lower than what they suggest. The key with any medication is to find the "sweet spot" for the individual, and we are usually not able to determine that until the person is treated, as we see the clinical results. These medications that I have listed were welcome additions to the armamentarium, but I was happy to see a new batch coming in that would be even better in certain ways.

The next batch of atypicals started around the time when Saphris (asenapine) came out in 2009, which was certainly an exciting medication to work with. None of them are perfect, but each has its advantages. I was excited when Latuda (lurasidone) came out in 2010 for schizophrenia (which also means for Bipolar I Disorder), but then it also got approval in 2013 for the treatment of bipolar depression, though I was already using it for that when it first came out. I was hearing a lot of buzz about Latuda (lurasidone) when it arrived on the scene, and it has certainly proven to be an important addition to this class and quickly became even more popular than Saphris (asenapine). It not only has antagonism of dopamine D2 but also serotonin 5HT2A and 5HT7 receptors. It is overall gentle and tends to be calming, but it is less sedating than the earlier ones, as was the case with Abilify (aripiprazole) and Geodon (ziprasidone). However, it is typically dosed in the evening and helps with sleep quality if needed. It also has a lower incidence of weight gain than such drugs as Geodon (ziprasidone) and possibly Saphris (asenapine). When weight gain is a concern, Latuda (lurasidone) has been my first choice for years, though since then there are other newer choices that also have a relatively low risk of this.

An interesting aspect of Latuda (lurasidone) is that if it is not taken with food, it is only half as effective. I usually dose it with dinner, but if it is sedating too early before bedtime, then it can be taken later with a snack of at least 350 calories, and if it is not, the company states that it is only half as effective. That's not a lot of food, so this should not be a problem since that's barely a snack (at least for me). One of the problems is that timing it with dinner can be difficult to remember since it is not a typical time that a medication is usually taken. If this is difficult to remember, I suggest that they set an alarm on their phone that goes off at the same time every day, which serves as a handy reminder. If they still can't remember to take it with food, I typically recommend that they double the dose in order to get the best efficacy. This may not always be needed, so we need to individualize this, and we should do this with everything that we do.

The next one of the newer atypicals that was released was Rexulti (brexpiprazole) in 2015, which was released by the company that sold Abilify (aripiprazole). I figured it would be a tweaking of the product, as was the case with previous newer medications, but I discovered that it was a completely different product that was distinct, and I was impressed with it right away when I started gaining experience with it.

As was the case with Abilify (aripiprazole), it's not usually sedating unless the dose is too high. Akathisia is something to watch for, though this is usually dosage dependent, as is the case with all of them in this class. The risk of akathisia from this medication, though, is less of a problem than with Abilify (aripiprazole). It also may lead to weight gain in certain individuals, as is potentially the case with Abilify (aripiprazole). Although this is an excellent medication, this is its biggest weakness.

I have found that the lower doses are better than the higher doses in most patients that benefit from it, which is not a surprise since that's also the case with all the others in this class. As was the case with Saphris (asenapine) and Invega (paliperidone), we were seeing overall better tolerance and better results than previous medications, though the older ones were still very effective and utilitous.

It was just so exciting when Rexulti (brexpiprazole) came out. It not only had dopamine and serotonin antagonism but also norepinephrine antagonism, thus providing the calming effect. It also has some dopamine and serotonin partial agonism of serotonin and norepinephrine, probably one reason that it is not usually sedating. Each one is a little different than the others, but that is what is so exciting about this class of medications. It is also effective for anxiety as well as depression, with, as I said, weight gain being the most common side effect, though it doesn't happen with every patient.

Rexulti (brexpiprazole) is marketed in a sense for treatment-resistant depression by advocating in these cases adding this product to an antidepressant to treat MDD when residual depressive symptoms persist in order to achieve remission. This has been a very successful strategy for many of my patients.

Here is also another interesting tidbit. It comes in 0.25 mg, 0.5 mg, 1 mg, 2 mg, 3 mg, and 4 mg. The dosage they recommend for augmentation for MDD is between 1 and 3 mg. In my experience 1 mg seems to be the most common dose, with 2 mg a close second. I never believed the sales line from the beginning. This does not behave like MDD at all. This is actually treating bipolar disorder and/or bipolar depression. I like to call it bipolar spectrum disorder. I first thought about the term "bipolar spectrum disorder" because I saw parallels with autistic spectrum disorder, which varies from mild to moderate to severe. Some of them are high-functioning, and some less so. Some of them are actually quite brilliant.

Here is the other most interesting part: Why would you have to add an atypical antipsychotic to the regimen to achieve improved results and possible remission? Atypical for MDD? It makes no sense. Obviously, this means that the person is in the bipolar realm and not in the unipolar realm. Here's the kicker: They market 1 to 3 mg for MDD and 4 mg for schizophrenia. Seriously? A 1 mg difference between MDD and schizophrenia? Really? It makes no sense.

The next one released in 2017 was Vraylar (cariprazine), which has a unique mechanism of action as compared to the other atypicals. The others focus mostly on D2, but Vraylar (cariprazine) affects D3 8:1 over D2 with serotonin antagonism but also acts as a partial agonist at serotonin and dopamine, which is probably why it is usually activating. It is formally indicated not just for schizophrenia at the highest dose of 6 mg, as is typically the case with all of the medications in this class, but more for bipolar mixed episodes, a combination of depression and mania or hypomania, so it is good in difficult cases, though all the others are also usually helpful for even the most difficult patients that we see. Balancing D3 may help with impulsivity such as OCD and other presentations, and it also has a decreased incidence of cognitive effects as compared to some of the others. It actually more likely seems to improve cognition.

Another advantage is that it is not typically sedating, but if it is, it can be taken at night. In most it is more likely activating/energizing. There is a potential for akathisia, as is the case with the others, but an advantage is that it doesn't typically lead to weight gain. I have found it very helpful for the more difficult-to-treat bipolar patients with mood fluctuations and swings as well as other more extreme presentations of both poles of bipolar disorder.

Vraylar (cariprazine) is also usually most helpful at the two lowest doses, with 1.5 mg being the most common dose, 3 mg the second most common, and the two higher doses less common. This is actually quite common among all of the atypicals. Unless we are dealing with the higher-grade versions, such as Bipolar I Disorder and possibly Bipolar II Disorder, it is commonly seen that the lower doses are best when it comes to Bipolar Depression. In the case of Vraylar (cariprazine), sometimes the lowest dose of 1.5 mg is too much, and it needs to be given every second or third day, sometimes even less frequently. This is because it has a long half-life. It is an effective and potent agent, and my only complaint is that it is a bit strong for some people. I wish that they would have come out with a 0.75 mg dose, which would make it easier to start and more easily tolerated at the beginning.

As is the case with Rexulti (brexpiprazole), they promote the lowest doses, especially the 1.5 mg dose, for treatment-resistant depression. In other words, it can be added to antidepressants in order to achieve remission. I have had a lot of success with this medication as the final piece or at least getting the person closer to remission. It makes no sense that we are treating difficult-to-treat MDD. Why would we need to add an atypical antipsychotic medication in order to treat unipolar disorder? What we are actually treating is bipolar depression or somewhere within the realm of bipolar spectrum disorder.

Even though I consider marketing Rexulti (brexpiprazole) and Vraylar (cariprazine) as augmenting agents to treat difficult-to-treat MDD as false advertising, there is a good side to them being marketed for this purpose. Many primary care providers are afraid of the "B word." They may either think that they don't see bipolar disorder or don't feel comfortable treating it. In actuality they definitely do see it even if they are not recognizing it, and they should learn to be comfortable treating it since the need is so desperate. Primary care providers are in the ideal situation to diagnose and treat these conditions because not only is the need so great, but the reality is that there are just not enough psychiatrists to be able to treat all that are in such desperate need of relief from their mental anguish. If they at least understand adding a mood stabilizer to an antidepressant is getting their patients better, hopefully at some point they will understand what they are actually treating and thus become more and more comfortable doing so. Hopefully this book, as well as my others, will help the cause.

One of the more recent atypical antipsychotics released is Caplyta (lumateperone). What confused me right off the bat was that they only released 42 mg sample tablets, which were touted as the starting and ending dose. I found this to be quite odd, since I had never seen this with the other atypicals. My initial experience with it was that it was not very well-tolerated, with the main problem being that it was too sedating the next day. Then a bit later I got 10.5 mg and 21 mg samples. This made much more sense to me since I like to start at the lowest dose and titrate to try to find the "sweet spot." Since then, my experiences with this product have been better, with some not needing the 42 mg dose. As I said, this was also the case with Vraylar (cariprazine) and is a common mistake from pharmaceutical companies. I think it is because they want efficacy to look good quickly in the studies, though it is important for doctors to understand that the lower and slower approach is usually best.

Lybalvi (olanzapine and samidorphan) is a combination of Zyprexa (olanzapine) and samidorphan, which is an opioid system modulator. This reduces the chance of weight gain, which is the biggest weakness of Zyprexa (olanzapine). However, one is not to take any opiate when taking this medication since it blocks its effects, which could increase the risk of overdose if one is taking an opiate.

The latest antipsychotic medication to come out at the time of this writing in 2025 is Cobenfy (xanomeline and trospium chloride). It is not listed as an atypical antipsychotic because it has a completely new and unique mechanism of action since it is not a dopamine D2 and serotonin antagonist. It is a muscarinic agonist at M1 and M4 in the brain while at the same time being an antagonist of muscarinic receptors in the peripheral tissue. This agonist–antagonist combination helps to make this a balanced medication. It is currently only indicated for schizophrenia, which is the case with many of the atypical antipsychotics when they are first released. I would predict that this medication will eventually come out with an indication for Bipolar I Disorder. This also may be the first in a new class of antipsychotics. It's exciting to see new and novel medications released to add to the psychotropic armamentarium.

The "Traditional" Mood Stabilizers

I tend to use the atypical antipsychotics more for mood stabilization, but we should not forget about the two "classic" ones. The mechanism of action of lithium carbonate is not completely known, but its therapeutic actions may be due to altered ion transport for inhibition of adenylyl cyclase, influencing nerve excitation, thus calming the brain. It is a tried-and-true effective medication, though there are some side effect issues to watch for, and we need to occasionally check kidney function, thyroid function, and lithium carbonate levels to check for toxicity or to see if the dose is too low and needs to be raised. In the literature it says that this product is good if someone has suicidal ideation; however, I believe that is the case with the other mood stabilizers also if the person has bipolar disorder.

Depakote enhances inhibitory neurotransmission of GABA and modulates voltage ion channels of calcium, as well as other actions that lead to calming of the brain. This is also a very effective medication, especially with the higher-grade bipolar disorders. It also requires occasional blood monitoring of Depakote levels to check for toxicity as well as the potential need to raise the dose. We also need to occasionally follow LFTs (liver function tests), but overall, this is a very safe and effective choice. It is a bit heavy-handed for some, but in many patients that I have had on this, the results can be excellent. I prefer the Depakote ER (divalproex sodium) form, which can be taken once a day in the evening in order to avoid sedation the next day. These classic mood stabilizers can be used together, and also one or both can be added to an atypical antipsychotic. Two or three mood stabilizers together are often a good approach for the more severe forms of bipolar disorders.

Lastly, Lamictal (lamotrigine) is a unique medication that has different mechanisms of action, with one being inhibition at the presynaptic level of glutamate. Since glutamate is the main excitatory neurochemical, this results in a calming of the brain. This is an excellent medication for bipolar depression and sometimes even helps the upper pole, not just the lower pole. This could be a good choice if one does not tolerate the typical antidepressants. It also can be added to one or more of them. In my experience, Lamictal (lamotrigine) is often the last piece of the puzzle if the patient is not in full remission or has a cyclical component.

We need to be careful when we are mixing Depakote with Lamictal (lamotrigine). Depakote interacts with it and increases the level of Lamictal (lamotrigine) in the system. This increases the risk of a serious dermatological emergency known as the Stevens-Johnson rash. In reality, however, the risk of this rash from Lamictal (lamotrigine) is extremely rare. I have been prescribing Lamictal (lamotrigine) for many years now, and I have never seen it happen even once. If the dosage increase causes any skin-related symptoms, I would simply lower the dose or stop it.

LET'S GO BACK IN TIME

I'd like to now take you back in time to my first Seroquel (quetiapine) and Seroquel XR (quetiapine ER) speaker training conference. As I said, I was confused as to why more doctors were not understanding my clinical experiences. It started to make more sense, though, when one of the speakers in a small group setting discussed that Bipolar Disorder comprises about 10% of Bipolar Disorder, Bipolar II about 20%, while 70% are classified as Bipolar Disorder NOS (Not Otherwise Specified). I questioned him as to why we were only discussing the most severe variation in the top 10% and not discussing the other 90%, but he said he couldn't really formally discuss that. The FDA only allowed them to discuss what it was originally indicated for, which was schizophrenia and Bipolar I Disorder.

As per usual, the initial dosing recommendations were way too aggressive, with starting the dose too high and titrating up the dose too quickly. I was starting at the lowest dose and titrating slowly and carefully as I closely monitored the results, since the low and slow approach is the best for most. The exception is for patients with more severe and acute mental illness requiring the highest of doses, so I could titrate up as quickly as it is needed, tolerated, and safe.

He and the other doctors in the room chuckled when I was questioning this because they knew that this was "off-label" information that was not supposed to be formally discussed, though I pointed out that it was only us there and that we should be able to speak more freely amongst ourselves. Though I shared my experiences, which received an enthusiastic reception, the lecturer quickly steered back to discussing only "on label" indications.

As I stated previously, free speech is a rarity when it comes to marketing and speaking about whichever psychotropic we are discussing. We are supposed to have the First Amendment right to free speech, right? The biggest problem is that if we are not allowed to speak freely with each other in order to exchange practical ideas, then most doctors will never understand the potential of the tools that we have so readily available at our fingertips. This is one of the many problems of having government involvement with the cutting-edge field of mind-body medicine. It's not a good mix. One of the reasons that I am so excited about writing and sharing these books is that I can speak freely if I am speaking for myself and my books and not for the pharmaceutical companies. I will then be able to speak freely about "off-label" ways that I do things that providers may not be able to hear anywhere else. This is the best approach in order for providers to really understand in depth how to approach the rational trial-and-error methods that are at the heart of The Corona Protocol.

During the Seroquel (quetiapine) and Seroquel XR (quetiapine ER) weekend conference, as well as with all the ones previously and since, we had to listen to a lecture about compliance, usually delivered by an attorney, discussing what we can and can't say. I've heard the lecture delivered in so many different ways by different attorneys that I could give the lecture myself by now. They basically tell us what is and isn't appropriate to say, which is in a sense offensive since the off-label information is really the good stuff. This is, in my opinion, just complete nonsense to not be able to discuss this subject more openly. I plan to do whatever it takes to try to change that. I believe it is more important to listen to and follow the advice of doctors rather than attorneys when it comes to a medical subject that is as cutting-edge as this is. I advise getting legal advice from attorneys and medical advice from physicians as a general rule.

I was able to get my message across to Dr., however, when I lectured since I spoke freely about whichever subject we were discussing. I would make it clear that this information was not from the company but rather from me and based on my personal experiences. I usually followed the prepared slide deck, which they wanted me to stick to, but I would elaborate in order to get the important information out.

My favorite was the question-and-answer period, when I would have the best opportunity to discuss the importance of prescribing it "off-label" and in what cutting-edge ways to use it. I would then, during this post-lecture time, be able to cover some areas that I wasn't able to fit in during the lecture. Back then there were many fewer restrictions on our free speech than there have been in recent years. Having more leeway gave me more opportunities to share the important things I had discovered. The restrictive regulations since then have just taken things way too far, to the point of ridiculousness. Given what we do for a living, we can handle the truth.

Another way I was able to get the word out was by welcoming the other doctors to come talk to me personally after the lecture, and then I would meet with them one-on-one. I gave out my cards so they could call me with any questions or if they would like to discuss any patient in particular. Unfortunately, most doctors just never get to hear this exciting information, either due to lack of interest or to the incomplete availability of information that they are exposed to at lectures, in journals, or in clinical practice. We need to be able to discuss freely all the exciting off-label and on-label ways prescriptions can be used.

As time passed, the compliance talks were getting more ridiculous in an attempt to squelch off-label information. Would we get in trouble? Not get paid? At one of the last speaker training conferences, we were told that we were to stick to the slide deck and not proactively discuss off-label information, as if it were dangerous. If off-label questions were asked during the Q&A section, we were told to meet with that person after the lecture so as to not subject the other doctors to off-label information. This is offensive to our sensibilities, treating us like children, as if off-label information was too dangerous of knowledge for us to be exposed to. I was disgusted and angry about this, since this was just going too far. This information is far too important to keep secret.

This obsession about the dangers of off-label information is not only the case with the atypicals but also the antidepressants and other mood stabilizers as well. I had wondered what the big deal was about discussing the myriad of benefits that psychotropics can provide and why they felt that this information would poison the minds of doctors by preventing the most cutting-edge information from reaching the prescribing physician. What was so threatening about this?

We know that with other medical problems that we treat, we often prescribe medications for other indications than just the original ones. That's just how we do things as clinicians. We learn as we go, and we find out along the way better ways and more creative ways to heal. So, what's the big deal? Why do the FDA and federal government care so much about this and make such an issue out of this? I really didn't get it back then, but I was determined to find out.

During Seroquel (quetiapine) and Seroquel XR (quetiapine ER) speaker training, I first heard a statistic that is the most shocking one I've ever heard in any field of medicine. It takes an average of 3 to 4 doctors (including psychiatrists) and 7 to 10 years in order to properly diagnose bipolar disorder. Think about that for a moment and let it sink in. Would it be acceptable to take that long and for many doctors, such as cardiologists and family physicians, to diagnose hypertension, high cholesterol, or heart disease? How about that many gastrointestinal or primary care doctors to diagnose acid reflux or peptic ulcer disease? How about oncologists for cancer? How many years and how many endocrinologists does it take to diagnose diabetes? Is there any other disease process that you can think of that would take that long and that many doctors to diagnose it? Of course not.

These examples would clearly be malpractice. So why is this acceptable? Why is there not widespread outrage about this? Because by and large doctors are not aware of this, and even if they are made aware, as when I lectured to the doctors about this, I'm not sure if much changed in their practices because of this knowledge as I had hoped. This statistic really shocked and confused me, but I was determined to find out why that was the case and what I could do about it.

Since in my next book, *The Corona Protocol Prescriber's Guide,* I list the formalized DSM-IV and DSM-5 definitions of the different types and varieties of bipolar disorder, and in my first three books, *Healing the Mind and Body: The Trilogy,* I discussed the subject also in further detail, I will not be repeating that information here. Rather, in this book I want to focus on the bigger picture. In the *Prescriber's Guide* I discuss the term "bipolar spectrum disorder," which is a term I really like because it implies that we are dealing with a disorder that has a full spectrum of presentations that have a lot of variety and subtleties that can be distinguished.

Bipolar I Disorder (and even more so Schizoaffective Disorder) is the higher-grade end of the spectrum, with Bipolar II more medium-grade, and Bipolar NOS (Bipolar III to VI or more) consists of more of the lower-grade to medium end of the spectrum.

Some of these patients are higher functioning, and some are lower functioning, and the majority are in-between, with lower- to mid- to higher-grade forms. In the case of bipolar disorder, we will be discovering more and more over time that there are so many subtle variations of this disorder left to explore along the spectrum.

Recognizing Bipolar Disorder

I will now review ways to recognize that we are dealing with the realm of bipolar disorder instead of unipolar disorder and other related diagnoses. There are many clues that we can look for in order to figure this out.

1) When Antidepressants Only Help So Much

Antidepressants are the cornerstone of treatment for unipolar disorder, but they also play an important role in bipolar disorder. In fact, the vast majority of bipolar patients, in my opinion, should be on at least one antidepressant, the rare exception being Bipolar I Disorder with mania and psychotic features, though even when that end of the spectrum is treated, many of them still require an antidepressant at some point in order to achieve full remission over the long haul. In some of those patients, however, mood stabilizers may be all that is needed. This is because mood stabilizers can help both poles of the spectrum since they have antidepressant effects as well as anti-mania and anti-hypomania effects.

Focusing back on depression though, many patients who appear to have unipolar disorder do not fully respond and achieve remission from antidepressants alone. A true unipolar patient should respond well and achieve remission with just antidepressants, and most patients need more than one to reach their goal. I will briefly review what I've covered in much more detail in previous writings.

There are four major classes of modern antidepressants (excluding the older MAOIs and tricyclic antidepressants): the SSRIs, the SNRIs, Wellbutrin, and Lamictal (lamotrigine). An SSRI or an SNRI is the usual first-line choice, and in my estimation SNRIs are better than SSRIs more than half of the time, probably 2/3 to 3/4 of the time. Wellbutrin is more rarely the best first-line choice, unless dopaminergic symptoms are dominant. Otherwise, it is usually better as an augmenting agent with an SNRI or an SSRI. It just happens to be the best augmenting agent available. The overall best combination, in my opinion, is the "Dynamic Duo," an SNRI-Wellbutrin combination, or less likely an SSRI-Wellbutrin combo, since Wellbutrin only balances norepinephrine slightly but often not enough.

Lamictal (lamotrigine) is an exciting medication and is a potential first-line choice for some, but more likely an augmenting agent for more difficult-to-treat, cyclical, or bipolar depression. However, for those who do not tolerate one of the typical antidepressants, Lamictal (lamotrigine) may be well. It can also be added to one or more of the more standard antidepressants. Lamictal (lamotrigine) is unique because it is both an antidepressant and a mood stabilizer at the same time.

A newer antidepressant, Auvelity (dextromethorphan/bupropion SR), is a powerful choice with a unique mechanism of action, with half of the medication, Wellbutrin SR, boosting dopamine and slightly norepinephrine, along with dextromethorphan, which boosts glutamate, which no antidepressant in the past has ever done. It is also a Sigma-1 alpha agonist, which modulates serotonin and norepinephrine. All of these actions make it a very unique and exciting new addition, the only new antidepressant that has come out in a while. This is a good choice for those with treatment-resistant depression. I typically try Wellbutrin XL first. If it does not give excellent efficacy or if the efficacy decreases over time, then switching to Auvelity (Dextromethorphan/Bupropion SR) is a good choice to consider for bipolar disorder even though it is an activating and powerful antidepressant. We just need to make sure that the patient is adequately mood stabilized in order to achieve the proper balance.

Deplin (L-methylfolate), Provigil (modafinil), or Nuvigil (armodafinil), and stimulants are more likely augmenting agents to add to the antidepressants for more complete results. That being said, what we often see is that no matter what antidepressant or combination of antidepressants that we put together, this only gets certain people so far. When this happens, it is very suspicious that bipolar spectrum disorder is at some level being uncovered, even without obvious "classic" signs of mania or hypomania. For difficult-to-treat cases we always need to keep in mind the possibility of a personality disorder.

The three mood-stabilizing choices are the atypical antipsychotics, the GABA/glutamate (anti-seizure) class, the "traditional" mood stabilizers lithium carbonate and Depakote, or a combination thereof. We have so many excellent choices in the exciting field of psychopharmacology.

We also have to be sensitive towards the psychological component, which may require counseling or other types of therapy, as well as the importance of a healthy lifestyle, including a regular cardiovascular exercise regimen, a well-balanced diet, and a healthy balance between work and play. Relaxation techniques such as learning to breathe properly, as well as meditation, yoga, contemplative prayer, and spiritual counseling, may also be invaluable.

The choice of which mood stabilizer depends on the history, symptoms, and presentation of the patient. I use the atypicals and GABA/glutamate classes more and reserve the "classics," lithium carbonate and Depakote, for more severe and treatment-resistant cases.

2) When Antidepressants Don't Work

It can be frustrating for the provider and patients if we think that we're treating unipolar disorder and they don't respond as they are supposed to. Didn't they read the manual? Anyway, if medications don't work, that may just mean that the correct neurochemical is not being addressed properly. There also may be an imbalance of more than one neurochemical, more often than not requiring more than just one antidepressant at a time.

It may be a combination of neurochemicals that are out of sync and require balancing. When even the "cocktails" don't work, though, it is time to reassess the situation and find out what is really going on. We need to assess if there is a history of trauma, PTSD, or other mood disorders. As I said, we also have to always keep in mind the possibility of one or more personality disorders, since psychotropic medications can take away the rough edges of the personality but cannot change the core personality traits.

Childhood trauma and abuse usually lead to more difficulty treating the condition adequately since there are mixed components that need to be addressed. Childhood sexual abuse is the most damaging of all, and it is very difficult for these patients to ever be fully healed. Emotional and physical abuse also can leave some deep scars that can be resistant to treatment. There is hope, though. EMDR therapy seems to be the most effective treatment for trauma and PTSD. The psychologist needs to be specially trained to do this.

If the patient does not respond to medication, it is necessary to reassess to determine if psychotherapy is potentially needed; this also involves assessing the patient's lifestyle habits, such as their exercise program, a well-balanced diet, and proper attention to relaxation techniques: meditation, yoga, and contemplative prayer. The other thing to keep in mind is that if the patient does not respond to antidepressants, then a subtle presentation of bipolar disorder may actually be the underlying cause, which means focusing our attention on mood stabilizers.

We also need to assess whether addiction is a significant part of the presentation, which makes treatment more challenging and resistant to being adequately treated. Addiction simply means that a patient is self-medicating an underlying mood disorder, whether it be depression, anxiety, bipolar disorder, or another mental health condition. Getting these patients to sobriety is the most important goal, with adequate psychological and medical help, which includes the proper use of psychotropic medications as well as attention to the general medical health of that individual.

3) When Antidepressants Worsen Mood

When this happens, I first remove the antidepressant and then reassess if I need to switch to a different antidepressant class. The right one should be well-tolerated, and the efficacy should be obvious. If not, it is probably the wrong one, or it may mean that the other antidepressants also will not be tolerated or won't work. If the patient gets worse with an antidepressant, then I reassess to see if the patient is more within the unipolar spectrum or bipolar spectrum. If we are leaning in the bipolar direction, then instead of an antidepressant, a mood stabilizer will more likely be a better choice. The reality, though, for most of these patients is that antidepressants and mood stabilizers combined together lead to the best results with just the right cocktail.

Sometimes the antidepressant will improve mood, such as depressive and anxiety symptoms, but lead to hypomania or mania. This unmasking of the bipolar component signals the next course of treatment. If the antidepressant leads to severe side effects such as over-activation and suicidal ideation, then the best course would be to stop the antidepressant as soon as possible. If the instability, however, is not that bad and the positive results are obviously seen, then a mood stabilizer can be quickly added in order to adequately stabilize the mood by tuning down the hypomania or mania symptoms.

Another option is to lower the antidepressant dose, since bipolar patients often need lower than average doses of antidepressants as compared to our unipolar patients. If the mood stabilizers are not adequately stabilizing mood, then it is better to stop an antidepressant and reassess if and when it is re-added, or we can decide if another one should be tried instead. This is where instinct and experience come in handy.

In a similar fashion, when mood stabilizers work their best, depression may be uncovered, often presenting with low motivation, low energy, and depressed mood. This usually signals the need to start an antidepressant or for the dose already taken to be increased, continued the same, or tried for potentially even better. If antidepressant doses are increased or after augmentation, then the mood stabilizers may need to be increased, and then vice versa. We need to learn how to tune up and tune down psychotropic medications appropriately when needed in order to get patients in the right rhythm and keep them in tune.

In general, if an SSRI is too activating, then this may mean that a more calming SSRI would be a good choice. It depends if the medication gives enough positive results to warrant certain side effects. If the patient's symptoms are more related to serotonin, then an SSRI or "super" SSRIs like Viibryd (vilazodone) and Trintellix (vortioxetine) may be the best option. In some it may mean that norepinephrine imbalance is a key component and that attempting to balance only serotonin leads to unsatisfying results. The risk of potential side effects can scare people away from trying something else that could help due to an irrational fear of side effects.

Some people are so fearful about side effects that it holds them back from trying medications that may help. I try to reassure nervous patients that side effects are not dangerous and typically mild, and if not, then the medication can be stopped or the dose can be lowered. Some bipolar patients are more sensitive when it comes to antidepressant side effects, and the antidepressant choice depends on whether norepinephrine is a factor or not. Some of the higher-grade bipolar patients may be extra sensitive to noradrenergic effects, and in these cases an SSRI would be better if serotonin is a key component and/or Wellbutrin if dopamine is a significant factor. It usually is in bipolar disorder, which is why Wellbutrin XL is such an attractive agent. The boosting effect of dopamine combined with an atypical antipsychotic, which is a dopamine antagonist. This combination is what I refer to as balancing dopamine 24/7, which is a powerful combination that I put together quite often. Wellbutrin XL is, in my opinion, the best augmenting agent that we have available. An excellent backup plan is Auvelity (dextromethorphan/bupropion SR), which boosts glutamate, dopamine, norepinephrine, and even serotonin a bit. It is a powerful tool that we now have available in the psychotropic toolbox.

If we decide to choose a trial of an SNRI, starting low and going slow can be the best way to tell whether a dual-action medication is needed. This can be both diagnostic and therapeutic at the same time. If an SNRI is too activating, though, or increases anxiety, this is a signal to stop it and reassess whether a different antidepressant is needed or three mood stabilizers instead. A potential good choice to consider in this situation would be Lamictal (lamotrigine), which is basically a combination of an antidepressant and mood stabilizer and is an excellent antidepressant choice in bipolar disorder.

There is a myth that patients with bipolar disorder should not be given SNRIs, though I have noticed that this is often not the case. Sometimes it just takes adequate mood stabilization to be able to tolerate the boosting of norepinephrine seen with an SNRI. However, in some of these patients an SSRI is better tolerated and may even have better efficacy, so it really depends on the individual that we are treating.

If the patient has schizoaffective disorder or a high-grade Bipolar I Disorder then we need to take greater care as to the antidepressant choice. These patients may not be the best candidates for an SNRI, unless the other antidepressant choices fail to deliver.

It often requires a lower dose of any of the antidepressants, except for Lamictal (lamotrigine), than a patient with unipolar depression. Contrary to popular opinion, SNRIs may be very efficacious in bipolar disorder, especially if there are somatic and/or anxiety symptoms remaining that are related to the depression as well as bipolar symptoms. It's difficult to beat the efficacy of an SNRI, so it really comes down to if it is tolerated adequately and is worth the results.

If we can recognize that a patient has bipolar disorder and if we are unsure whether to treat with an antidepressant or mood stabilizer, it's probably safer to start with a mood stabilizer, especially if there are hypomanic or manic symptoms predominating, such as the higher-grade bipolar variants with signs of instability.

The lower-grade presentations of bipolar disorders are best defined as bipolar spectrum disorder, with the lower grades being dominated by depressive symptoms that can be persistent and difficult to treat. In these cases, we focus on antidepressants, though mood stabilizers are helpful as augmentation at some point. Mood stabilizers also have antidepressant properties, and there is a symbiotic effect on mood between the antidepressants and mood-stabilizing classes.

However, when it comes to treating depressive symptoms, antidepressants are the gold standard, even if there is a bipolar component. These patients may need lower doses of mood stabilizers and also may be able to handle more average doses of the antidepressants than those at the higher end of the spectrum. We figure out as we treat patients what doses of antidepressants and mood stabilizers it takes in order to optimally treat all the different aspects of mood as it relates to the body. When the final mix is in place and we see the results, then we can figure out exactly what type of mood disorder that we are dealing with whatever we are presented with and learn to do it the best we can.

This may sound strange to some, but side effects actually help us to know if we are treating correctly or not. Most side effects are not severe and are tolerable, so it can then be assessed whether they are worth it depending on what the positive results are. By balancing positive results with side effects, it can then be determined as to how to increase or lower medications in the right combination in order to maximize the positive results and minimize the negative effects at the same time.

Optimizing efficacy and minimizing side effects by using the rational trial-and-error polypharmaceutical approach is the cutting-edge way to treat these disorders. This involves learning from our mistakes, since when it comes to science, practice makes perfect, with the goal of full remission for all of the patients that trust us with their care.

4) When Mood Is Cyclical

In order for my methods and protocol to work, it is of vital importance that we take a complete history and observe all the details that are provided. We need to observe how mood has changed over time and if it changes in any cyclical fashion or not. It can be subtle for some, though the instability often follows certain patterns. For example, some patients have a cyclical change every few months or so, with rapid cycling defined as four episodes or more per year. For some it happens more often and for others less often. Some cycles are subtle, while others are more obvious. We can learn how to predict the future by learning from the past by taking a very detailed past history.

In order to recognize when cycling happens, we need to take as complete and detailed of a history as we can, with every nuance of the history appreciated, recognizing both emotional and physical symptoms as they relate to the mood and to the body. We need to explore the different stages of life, such as childhood, adolescence, early adulthood, midlife, and the elder years, documenting each significant event that alters the course along the way. We need to document when the patient has had depressive symptoms, anxiety symptoms, mania, and hypomania, as well as physical symptoms.

In order to gauge what normal is, I ask every new patient when he or she felt the best in life and when that changed. Understanding the details of these changes is the key to proper diagnosis and treatment. The most common times people say they felt their best were in childhood, such as in elementary school, before puberty and in middle school. This is often a more carefree time of life, as long as one is raised in a nurturing and loving environment free of any form of abuse.

Not everyone has a "Mayberry" upbringing as many of us had. For some it can be a time of neglect as well as emotional and/or physical abuse, which can contribute obviously to what kind of mood that person is in. Growing up in fear and in pain is not a good foundation to build upon. The scars left due to the abuse are difficult to heal, especially sexual abuse before puberty, though this of course affects one at any age.

Many have difficulty ever getting past the abuse and damage from the past, though with adequate counseling, time, and the proper treatment plan, such as The Corona Protocol, they have a good chance of being helped and ultimately healed. The best type of psychotherapy to treat any type of abuse and trauma is EMDR therapy, which is a specialized form that the psychologist needs to be trained to learn how to do.

The other time of life when people state that they felt their best and felt like themselves is the late teens into the early-to-mid-20s. It is rare for people to say that middle school to high school were the best years of their life. Puberty and the teenage years can be a rocky time since these years are a time of changing neurochemical imbalances when hormones are radically changing. This is one of the most stressful times for people, along with middle age, which we will discuss in a bit.

Getting out of high school and moving on in life can be a fearful time for some, but it can also be an exciting time to be independent and explore the future with hope and excitement. Some people go to college, graduate school, and beyond. Some start training through trade school, where they learn their craft. This time of life is also a time to be single and free, waiting until a bit later in life for marriage and children when the time is right. However, for some that is not the case. For some the happiest time of life is when they have children and raise them. Whichever time of life is "normal" for that person, then I do what we need to make that a reality again.

Some people have had horrible upbringings and life experiences in childhood or in their 20s, and so they may not understand what feeling "normal" really means. I enjoy watching people find out what normal really feels like and how we can achieve and sustain that in the future. Once neurochemicals are properly balanced, then we can experience what a healthy "normal" really can be.

For some the best times are the teenage years or the 30s, 40s, or beyond, though when life gets more complicated, it becomes less carefree, with more work and less fun. For some, though, the happiest time is having children and raising them. Whichever time of life is at its happiest and most normal is the goal that we are striving for, getting them back to their old selves or better than that, depending on the individual. Feeling normal means feeling happy and having a balanced, functional, fun, and joyful life. There are so many people desperately in need of this type of true inner happiness.

When mood changes and shifts either daily, weekly, monthly, or cyclically throughout the year, this is highly predictive of a bipolar component of the disorder. It could, of course, also mean that the wrong antidepressant is being given if it destabilizes the mood, and in this case, we can then assess whether a different antidepressant or a mood stabilizer is the best next step. Once we get the mix right, even if we get to full remission, it is possible in some that this won't last and the mood will crash at some point. This may not be as bad as the original poor mood, or in some cases it can be worse. We then can assess whether to increase the dose, change the antidepressant, and add or tweak a mood stabilizer.

If the efficacy was good, though, I would typically continue the course and add something that will help resolve the cycling. If the results are partial, then we can assess whether to change the antidepressant to a potentially better one or if it should be continued as is and focus instead on a mood stabilizer as an augmenting agent.

If the patient has bipolar depression or if the patient is in the depressive cycle of bipolar disorder, Lamictal (lamotrigine) can be an excellent choice, since if glutamate is a factor and moving too quickly through the nervous system, then this medication suppresses glutamate and thus calms the brain and central nervous system. A newer antidepressant, Auvelity (dextromethorphan/bupropion SR), boosts dopamine and norepinephrine with half of it being Wellbutrin SR, as well as boosting glutamate and even a little serotonin with the other half. It is indicated for unipolar depression and treatment-resistant depression and not bipolar depression; however, it still may be useful as long as the person is adequately mood stabilized.

In bipolar patients, Lamictal (lamotrigine) may be the only antidepressant needed, especially for the higher-grade bipolar patients. It really just depends on the reaction to the more first-line usual antidepressants or if the patient has a higher grade of bipolar disorder and thus is more sensitive to SSRIs, SNRIs, or even Wellbutrin.

Lamictal (lamotrigine) can also be an augmenting choice to add to the other antidepressants if there is still a cyclical and depressive nature to the mood. It can also help reduce mania or hypomania to a lesser degree than its effect on depression, so it is a true mood stabilizer and antidepressant at the same time.

That is also the case with the atypical antipsychotics, the other GABA agents, and the traditional mood stabilizers. These focus more on the higher-end symptoms such as mania or hypomania but also have antidepressant effects.

The correct diagnosis and optimal treatment plan can be elusive for many, leading to under-recognition and under-treatment of very treatable conditions. It's easier, though, than we may initially think, and this requires interest in the ability to feel comfortable practicing with the rational trial-and-error method until we get the treatment just right for each individual. The error part, though, gets less and less as we practice until we get it right more quickly and consistently.

Mood cycles sometimes can have a usual pattern, while others are unpredictable. This may vary with the stressors going on at the time, but sometimes there is a separate seasonal component that is predictive. The most common time in general for depression is the holiday season. During that time the days are shorter because it gets dark earlier, and that decreased amount of sun time means that it gets dark at or soon after the end of the workday. It is well documented that areas with less sunshine, more rain, and more overcast days result in an increased risk of depression. When it's colder and darker, the mood tends to follow suit.

The "Holiday Blues" is very common due to uncovering memories of both the good and bad of our past and our family. It is a unique time of reflection on our past and contemplation about our future. Many people remember losses of loved ones during this time. Some family members come together even when, in some cases, they probably shouldn't. They may not see each other much the rest of the year, and remember why that is the case. If we force people together that probably really shouldn't be together because they don't like each other, this can lead to dysfunction and conflict, thus sabotaging the family get-together and creating bad memories for all.

For many though, such as myself, the holiday season is the happiest time of year, when the weather cools down, the holiday music starts playing, the holiday food and drinks are served, parties start happening, family rituals are followed (like our tamale making for our annual Christmas Eve party for family and friends at our house), people are more generous, and holiday cheer is the rule. Fall to winter is also my favorite sports season and the only one I'm interested in, college football, featuring the USC Trojans and the Nebraska Cornhuskers.

We need to keep track of which seasons lead to which type of mood shifts, either depressive, manic, or hypomanic, or a combination thereof. Patients may experience hypomania and mania in the spring and summer, which can eventually lead to depression. This depression is the state most common in bipolar disorder, is typically worse than the depression experienced in unipolar disorder, and carries an increased risk of suicidal thinking and behaviors. Once we see the individual's pattern, then we're more ready with the most helpful treatment course, which leads to the correct cures that last throughout the year.

One way of distinguishing bipolar disorder is the depth and complexity of the mood state. The depression is typically deeper and more resistant to treatment. It is more complex in its nature, and its presentation is more dramatic and more of a challenge to resolve. When people think of bipolar disorder, mania is the foremost symptom one thinks of; hypomania is less recognizable and understood, even though it happens more often than mania does. That's one main reason that doctors miss this diagnosis so much, because they are focused on the upper pole but not the lower one. It is common to misdiagnose hypomania as anxiety. In bipolar disorder, depression is often more severe and intractable, and because people spend most of their time in this state, it is often misdiagnosed as unipolar disorder by so many doctors. It is crucial to understand this, since not doing something about it is the key reason why bipolar patients don't get fully better.

If we take an adequate history, we should be able to meter out the difference by looking at the pattern of the disorder over time, which is more unstable and more resistant to treatment. When the depression does not respond to antidepressants the way we think that it should, it's time for us to reconsider the diagnosis. If the condition is not quickly responding to unipolar agents or a combination of them, or is getting worse, this is suspicious, and we need to change course. A mood stabilizer at this point can make all the difference in the world, since it can redirect our attention to treating it in a newer and better way, which usually requires antidepressants also in order to complete treatment correctly. We figure this out as we follow the patient over time and as we intervene accordingly depending on the patient's presentation.

Antidepressants may improve the mood or rather may destabilize the patient, leading to mania or hypomania, while mood stabilizers may stabilize the mood but leave residual symptoms of depression. Following these cyclical changes until they even out and stop happening is the ultimate goal of treating cyclical mood disorders, helping our patients to be in control of their lives throughout the year by balancing all of the neurochemicals needed most properly depending on the needs of each individual in order to restore proper homeostasis for each of our clients and friends.

5) When Mood Disorders Occur Early in Life

If a person has a significant imbalance of mood early in life, especially before puberty, then this is a hint that there is or eventually will be a bipolar component to the mood presentation. As I said before, childhood is supposed to be the most carefree time of life when one doesn't have a lot of responsibilities and worries. It's supposed to be just about having fun and playing, before life gets more serious and complicated as we get older.

Some are fortunate to have loving and nurturing parents, while others are not so fortunate. Those who are exposed to significant emotional and physical abuse have more of a likelihood of developing a significant mood disorder, since these patients have more of a likelihood of having a significant genetic load passed down to the child given the parents' behaviors and actions. Both nurture and nature are involved, here, especially.

Children exposed to sexual abuse have the worst prognosis, since it is very difficult to ever get over that type of trauma. Physical, emotional, and mental abuse, as well as neglect, are also quite damaging to the victim. The good news is that even if someone has a significant disorder such as depression, anxiety, OCD, PTSD, ODD (oppositional defiant disorder), conduct disorder, bipolar disorder, or ADD/ADHD, treatment can be challenging. Nonetheless, it is still quite treatable—and potentially curable—the majority of the time.

The presentation may be unipolar at the beginning, but then the mood may switch over time. Prepubescent children who have significant presentations of their mood are more likely to fall along the bipolar spectrum rather than the unipolar spectrum. This will likely change when puberty occurs during middle school going into high school, the dreaded teenage years. This can be a very rocky time as well as a very fun time for many, and sometimes teenagers don't have the maturity and foresight to make the best choices and decisions.

6) When the Teenage Years Are More Dysfunctional Than Usual

The onset and completion of puberty during the middle school to high school years can be a rocky road for some. This is a time of potential high-risk behaviors such as drinking and drug use and is a time for sullen dispositions and moodiness. However, when the symptoms and onset are more extreme and dramatic, that may be suspicious of a bipolar element, especially if there is a history of onset in childhood. The more unstable the mood, the more severe the addictive behaviors can be, and the higher-risk behaviors can occur. This can then potentially lead to early sexual experiences, potentially with multiple partners due to hypersexuality, which may be drug-fueled and associated with mania or hypomania. Those with more irritable and angry moods, and those with extreme highs and lows, are all clues that they are within the bipolar spectrum.

This is especially evident as we start treating it and seeing how it responds to our medication choices. The teenage years can be so turbulent due to a combination of genetic factors, hormonal changes, previous diagnoses, poor impulse control, immaturity, narcissism, and a variety of other factors. This can also be a very happy time when it is done in a healthy way, and this also can be an exciting time as they plan their future education and career. The healthier our teenage experience, the more likely that we will become functional and happy adults. Even when the teenage years are rocky, that doesn't mean it's not going to get better, because thankfully even the most difficult patients that we see are fully treatable if done in the right way.

7) Genetics

Getting a detailed family history is extremely important, since we can get a lot of clues as to what diagnosis we are dealing with. If one has a milder family history, and especially if there is only a significant history on one side, then it is possible that the problem is unipolar disorder, whereas those who have stronger family histories, especially on both sides, are more likely to be in the bipolar spectrum. Those with "loaded" family histories and who respond to my inquiry about their family history with "How much time do you have?" answer the question as to how strong the genetic factors are.

When studying a family history, I look at the most immediate relatives, such as siblings, parents, grandparents, aunts and uncles, cousins, etc. I note if there is a family history of schizophrenia, bipolar disorder, suicide, depression, anxiety disorders, or nervous breakdowns; whether there is an addiction problem with alcohol and/or other illicit drugs, psychiatric hospitalizations, and other obvious clues.

What may not be as obvious are people who lead erratic and dysfunctional lives, those who move frequently, those in and out of relationships quickly, those who have had multiple marriages, and other signs of dysfunction and instability. They tend to have high highs and low lows and can be difficult to be around. If there is a strong family history on both sides, then the odds are against that person.

With the "old school" mentality, our ancestors typically would not share personal and family secrets that were hush-hush, meaning not shared readily with children and grandchildren, making it difficult to know. They often didn't like to talk about personal information and certainly not emotions. It was just a different mentality back then, so it can be difficult to get them to accept treatment in a way that they were not used to. There was a sense of pride and shame and not wanting to display signs of weakness, which is especially the case with men, which is why it is more difficult to convince them to be treated. We cannot help that there are genetic factors, but that doesn't mean we can't do something about it.

Strong clues include "My mother is a nervous lady" or "My father drinks too much and gets angry and mean." This usually means that she has an anxiety disorder and probably some depression, and that father was probably an alcoholic with an underlying mood disorder with anger issues that he was self-medicating. Either of them may have at least Bipolar Spectrum Disorder, causing irregularity of mood, and these mood disorders can also increase the chance of self-medicating, which can lead to addiction. Even though many of our relatives were never formally diagnosed, it's still obvious when we get a good family history that something significant was going wrong with them.

It can also be helpful to ask patients which parent or other relative they take after most with regard to personality, looks, and temperament. Even though we inherit genetics from both parents and both sides of the family, the patient has a higher risk of having whatever mental illness and addiction risk that those more closely resembling relatives have struggled with. I realize that we get stuff from both parents, but still there is usually one side of the family with whichever individuals we have the most in common with by sharing certain characteristics.

Genetic predisposition, though, does not mean that the person is necessarily predetermined to follow the same path, though the risk is certainly higher. There are other factors to keep in mind, though, such as a person's upbringing, coping skills, support system, and learning to make better choices, as well as other factors.

However, even if the person has a healthier situation, the person with a strong family history is just more at risk for having problems. There's also the fact that the person who is raised by emotionally unhealthy parents has more difficulty avoiding following similar unhealthy patterns. The apple may not fall far from the tree. The good news, though, is that once genetic factors are identified, the risks can be reduced and resolved with proper recognition and treatment.

8) Addictions

People become addicted to substances for various reasons. Many people can drink alcohol responsibly and are even able to do certain drugs recreationally without developing a dependence. It really boils down to if the patient is "self-medicating" a mood disorder in order to escape reality and forget about their problems if they are unhappy with their situation.

Some people fall into addiction due to peer pressure and hanging out with the "wrong crowd," especially during the adolescent and teenage years. If someone is drinking or doing drugs to wind down after work or in order to calm anxiety, sleep, and slow down the racing brain, the use of whichever substance is more likely to become a problem. If someone needs to do street drugs or drink in order to function and just to get through their day, this is a real problem.

Over 50% of patients with bipolar disorder struggle with addiction, definitely a higher risk than patients who have unipolar disorder, though they also have a high risk if it is not treated correctly. Addiction, simply put, is a brain disease and a true mental health crisis. This is also the case with other mood disorders, and it is not coincidental that a poor mood leads to addiction and addiction leads to a poor mood. This creates a true vicious cycle that is difficult to break.

Even though some people can experiment with "soft core" substances, such as alcohol, THC, and tobacco, and not become addicted and dependent, for others these can be a "gateway" to the more "hard core" drugs like heroin, methamphetamines, cocaine, hallucinogens, nitrous oxide, "party" drugs like Ecstasy and others, high doses of minor tranquilizers/benzodiazepines, opiates/pain pills, kratom, etc. Those who fall into a heavy addiction pattern are more likely the bipolar patients, while those who struggle less may be more likely to be unipolar.

When I get an addiction history, I ask patients what they like about certain drugs, as this can give me clues as to which medications might be the best for that individual. Psychotropic medications treat these conditions preventatively in a non-addictive way rather than the reactive way, which focuses on symptomatic medications that can become problematic. We should rather focus on optimal prevention, which is totally achievable. Once prevention is optimized with the proper psychotropic medications, this then leads to a decreased need for symptomatic medications and other forms of self-medicating, which is a much healthier preventative approach.

The term "dual diagnosis" (addiction along with mental illness), I believe, is an underappreciated term. In my opinion the vast majority of people who struggle with addiction also have an underlying mood imbalance that strongly contributes. The addiction part can be successfully treated with rehab facilities, sober living environments, AA, NA, and other 12-step meetings, individual counseling, group counseling, spiritual counseling, and other ways. The reason, though, that many attempts at sobriety fail, in my opinion, is that the underlying mood disorder is underappreciated and undertreated. Many have not been treated correctly or not at all. For these reasons, this is why, in my opinion, the relapse happened so frequently, along with cross-addiction to something else, whether it be nicotine, gambling, sexual and/or porn addiction, or other addictive substances and behaviors.

There is unfortunately an "anti-pill" mentality in the sobriety community, even for nonaddictive psychotropic medications, such as antidepressants and mood stabilizers. I believe this is the main issue that leads to such common relapsing after achieving sobriety. Under-treating or not treating the underlying mood disorder at all is the very reason why the addiction developed in the first place. Until this issue is truly appreciated, frequent relapsing will continue to be the norm.

It's certainly not 100% that even if someone's mental illness is well treated that they still won't fall back into unhealthy patterns, but it certainly improves their odds dramatically if they are healthy and happy with the use of the amazing and nonaddictive psychotropic medications that we have so readily available. It is certainly nice to have so many good choices. We just need to learn to appreciate them and use them properly.

9) Chaotic Lifestyles

I already alluded to this, but people with bipolar disorder tend to lead much more unstable lives in general as compared to those with unipolar disorder. They tend to have more problems with interpersonal relationships, have more problems with their bosses and coworkers, tend to move more frequently and change jobs more frequently, get married and divorced more often, have affairs more often, have problems with gambling and other addictive behaviors such as tattoos and piercings, tend to have more plastic surgery, have more financial problems due to poor decision-making, and more frequently struggle with addiction and have more difficulty staying in sobriety.

They also have more run-ins with the law. Our prisons are, in my opinion, the largest psychiatric wards that we have available. The vast majority of prisoners suffer from some form of mental illness. Common conditions include bipolar disorder, schizophrenia, and personality disorders like psychopathy and sociopathy. Many also have untreated and often self-medicated ADD/ADHD, along with depression and anxiety disorders that contributed to their poor choices.

Bipolar patients tend to have more problems at home getting along with family members and relatives and can cause chaos, turmoil, and emotional drain. They are more likely to say mean and hurtful things that they later regret (or not), since when they are in a manic state, they are not rational and thus make irrational decisions and statements when they are not thinking clearly due to a mood disorder, addiction, or a combination of both.

They're more likely to get into physical and verbal altercations with the spouse, children, siblings, parents, and even their friends. They are far more likely than unipolar patients to have the police called to intervene about a domestic disturbance. They are likely to be easily prone to violence with whoever is in their lives, and this can even result in run-ins with the law. They are very unstable individuals.

When they are out of the manic or hypomanic state and fall into depression, it can be a deep and morbid state, which can tend to draw in those around them since their sadness can be so all-encompassing. They may have regrets about their actions when they were in a manic state, which heightens the sadness. The apologies, though, can fall on deaf ears if this is a repetitive pattern and the person goes back to doing the same destructive behaviors when they are out of the depressive state. This is a pattern that can go on and on if not broken by paying full attention to all the details that lead to possibly healing the mind and body in order to lead them into full remission.

10) Insomnia

The majority of patients with bipolar disorder have problems with sleep. Unipolar patients often struggle with insomnia also, but it tends to be easier to treat and not as severe. People with anxiety disorders often have more difficulty getting to sleep, while those with depressive disorders are more likely have early-morning awakenings and then difficulty getting back to sleep.

Bipolar patients, though, often have problems with both, with difficulty getting to sleep due to racing thoughts and a highly active mind, and with difficulty shutting it down at night. Unipolar patients are more likely to respond to OTC and herbal remedies as well as prescription sleeping pills and lower-dose tranquilizers, while bipolar patients often need higher doses of sleeping pills and tranquilizers, and even that often doesn't work very well.

Unipolar patients often have their insomnia resolved with the proper use of antidepressants and preventative antianxiety agents, while bipolar patients will need heavier medications such as mood stabilizers to best help with sleep, such as the atypical antipsychotic class (with Seroquel (quetiapine) and Seroquel XR (quetiapine ER) often the best of the bunch) and the GABAergic medications. It's much better for the patient to focus on these non-addictive solutions rather than relying on high doses of tranquilizers and sleeping pills, which are not only addictive but also can exacerbate the problem by not treating the underlying cause and only focusing on the symptoms. This is what happens when we focus on symptomatic and reactive care rather than preventative and curative care.

Another way to distinguish the insomnia related to bipolar disorder is that these patients often feel a decreased need to sleep. This is the case with the hypomania of Bipolar II Disorder: they function fine the next day with little sleep. It is even worse with the mania of Bipolar 1 Disorder when they can't shut the brain down and can go days or even weeks with no or little sleep and are still able to somehow function. Unipolar patients rather feel very tired the next day if they don't get a good night's sleep, and that is also the case for some bipolar patients, however, some of them feel that a few hours' sleep is all they need, and then they are good to go the next day. They may feel that they are most productive at night when it is quiet and there are fewer distractions. It is very difficult for them to stop thinking and shut down their active brains.

Unipolar patients may toss and turn during the night when they are struggling to get back to sleep, while bipolar patients will more likely get up and get on the computer, watch TV, eat, and try to use the time productively (or not).

Bipolar patients tend to self-medicate more in order to sleep with alcohol, THC, and tranquilizers, often at higher dosages and quantities than unipolar patients.

Taking a good sleep history is invaluable when trying to assess what the correct diagnosis is so that proper treatment can begin, and the patient then has the hope that they will finally be able to achieve a healthy sleep pattern.

11) Personality Disorders

This is an endlessly fascinating subject. Chapter 6 of my second book on "Personality Disorders" is one of my favorite chapters of my first few books, *Healing the Mind and Body: The Trilogy*, since there is a variety of interesting personality types. There are plenty of details in that chapter, so I will focus on honing it down to the most important characteristics of the disordered personality types. Having a pathological problem with one's personality does not necessarily mean that the patient has bipolar disorder, but it certainly increases the odds.

Some patients with unipolar disorder, though, also have an accompanying personality disorder. It depends on how severe it is. If it is mild and the patient is functional, there is hope, because maybe he or she can then do what they can to try to change what is needed on their own or with therapy. Sometimes psychotropic medications help to balance previously imbalanced neurochemicals and thus get to the core of the problem and resolve the underlying cause of a disordered mood, whether depression, anxiety, mania, hypomania, ADD/ADHD, or a combination thereof. When they are treated correctly and thus have a better mood, their personalities tend to normalize somewhat, but rarely completely.

Maximizing nonaddictive antidepressants, mood stabilizers, and other supplements in whichever way needed provides the most complete results, treating in a preventative way rather than in a reactive way. Just treating the symptoms and not getting to the underlying core issue is, in my opinion, the wrong approach. Treating the mind and body at the same time just makes sense and leads to surprisingly amazing results consistently, with full remission possible for most everyone. However, there is a reason that I refer to them as "The Impossible Disorders," though there are exceptions to the rule.

Learning how to balance the nervous system properly so that the mind and body are in proper balance requires the rational trial-and-error polypharmaceutical approach, which leads to the best balance mentally, emotionally, and physically. Psychotropic medications can take away the rough edges and more extreme behaviors associated with personality disorders. When one feels better, one may be more able to control some of the negative aspects of the personality type.

Some patients feel more in control by reducing the physical and emotional symptoms at the same time with the use of certain antidepressants and mood stabilizers. It is much more common for individuals with a personality disorder to also have an underlying mood component, such as symptoms of depression, anxiety, bipolar disorder, or bipolar spectrum symptoms. If we treat mood disorders and personality disorders at the same time, then we can achieve the best outcomes. This is easier said than done, though, since the personality is really the core of that person, which can be very difficult to change.

I: Narcissistic, Histrionic, and Borderline (Cluster B)

Among the most common and most impactful types of disordered personalities are narcissistic, histrionic and borderline. The narcissist is all about himself or herself, not caring for others nearly as much as he cares for himself. They are very self-centered and tend to have very little regard for the feelings of others. They always think that they're right and that they are smarter and cleverer than you. Most narcissists are men, though it can also happen to women at times. They tend to have low self-esteem, though you may not know that due to the bravado. They are typically grown adults acting like children, with an obvious lack of maturity and insight, as well as with poor impulse control.

The histrionic personality is more often seen in women, and they are all about drama. They like to create a scene in which they get all the attention that they crave. They act way more dramatically than the situation warrants. I've seen them labeled as "drama queens" who thrive on crisis and love the attention. They are highly emotional, and their moods go up and down. This can also coexist with the narcissistic personality. When we combine the poor mood with a disordered and unhealthy personality, this can really lead to significant problems that are not always easy to fix.

The dramatic and over-the-top presentations are characteristic of histrionics, with hypochondriacal fears about the physical symptoms they are having and thinking they are in poor health when in reality they are usually healthy. It's very common for all the diagnostic tests to be normal, but they still worry that something has been missed. Their presentations can be dramatic or more subtle, and their fears are often over-the-top and irrational.

The borderline personality is one of instability. People describe needing to "walk on eggshells" around them. They're not sure if it's going to be a good day or a bad day or somewhere in-between. Their moods are very up and down and sideways, and it can be like a roller coaster around these people. Their moods can swing rapidly, and they can get suicidal at times and cause self-harm to their bodies. They are attention seekers and like to make a scene at times, like the histrionics. This is more common in women than men, though still common in both.

Sometimes people have characteristics of two or three of these disordered personalities at the same time, which is even more challenging to treat and just to deal with in general. Some of them have a triple presentation, such as the narcissistic, histrionic, borderline patient. These are among the most challenging to treat, and I suggest that until they are adequately treated, the people in their lives keep a safe distance from these toxic individuals as much as possible in order to protect themselves. Those with disordered personalities usually do not have much insight into themselves.

At some point they need to change if they are going to get better. If they have the true desire to change and will put the work into it, then there is hope. If we work together, then we will potentially see good results at some point. The most effective type of psychotherapy for BPD is DBT (Dialectical Behavioral Therapy), which is very involved, and thus the reason that most people with this disorder don't actually take advantage of this therapy.

II: Avoidant, Dependent, Obsessive-Compulsive, Passive-Aggressive (Cluster C)

There is also a group of personality disorders that are less dramatic and yet still negatively impact others around them. If you work with them or otherwise know them, you may still be in some way impacted by the way they just are. They are the avoidant, dependent, obsessive-compulsive and the passive-aggressive.

The avoidant personality type presents as shyness to the extreme. They feel inadequate and are hypersensitive to criticism by others. They have low self-esteem and self-worth, are uncomfortable around others, and others may feel uncomfortable around them. It's difficult to get close to them.

The dependent personality type is someone who needs to be taken care of by someone else. They look to others to make decisions for them. They fear being abandoned and alone. They have few friends, except the ones that they depend on. People view them as needy and clingy, and people don't usually want to be around that kind of negativity. This may be cultural in certain societies where women are subservient and dominated by males. This is less likely in Western cultures and more likely elsewhere around the world. Other examples abound in our society when dependents of the government and the "welfare mentality" become chronic and a generational problem that is not easily fixable unless the issue is forced, which can then lead to the cycle being broken.

The obsessive-compulsive personality type can be extremely orderly and obsessive about specific ways of doing things. They can be high-strung, stressed out, inflexible, and have difficulty relaxing. They are often preoccupied with orderliness and neatness. Think Felix Unger in The Odd Couple. They can be very good and efficient employees, though they can come across as obnoxious and difficult to work with at times due to their inflexibility.

There are more males that have this personality disorder than females. Some of them have OCD with uncontrollable rituals and compulsive desires, though many may still have the strong personality traits without actual OCD. They usually benefit, though, from the use of psychotropic medications if they can be talked into it, and not just a traditional OCD medication like a high-dose SSRI. Some of them may be along the bipolar spectrum and thus need augmentation in order to get them feeling their best.

It's very difficult to change this personality type since it is so ingrained (as is the case with the other personality disorders), but sometimes medications take away the rough edges of the personality and mellow the person out. This is a very difficult personality to change, even with therapy, because he is stuck in his ways and usually doesn't really think he has a problem and needs to change. He may feel very comfortable with his obsessions and compulsions because he feels that this is just who he is.

The passive-aggressive personality type is not actually a "formal" personality disorder, as is the case with the others, but I discuss it here since it is still significant. It is characterized by a persistent pattern of creating the impression of active compliance with the others while subtly resisting them at the same time. They are the backstabbers who pretend they are on your side while undercutting you at the same time. They can be stubborn and sullen and make excuses as to why something was not done. They are manipulative and tend to shift the blame to others. They may be obnoxious and can be difficult for others to be around. They like to stir up trouble.

They often have underlying mood disorders, which can be successfully treated; however, the personality is much more difficult to change. They often don't see themselves as the problem and don't then see the need to change, so the person will likely stay the same in the future.

Counseling with this group of disordered personalities can definitely help if the person is receptive and desires to make healthy changes. As with the others, medications can at least take away the rough edges of the personality and mellow it out so they may then be easier to be around. This can help them heal relationships when they are more in control. Often though, no matter how good the medications are, and even with therapy, the underlying personality type of the person rarely truly changes, unless they want to change and think they need to change, which unfortunately is rare.

III: Paranoid, Schizoid, and Schizotypal (Cluster A)

The next group of personality disorders I will discuss are stranger and more bizarre than the previous ones and are also more dysfunctional for the person than those around them. They may come across as strange and eccentric, though they are usually harmless. They are the paranoid, schizoid and schizotypal.

The paranoid personality disorder is characterized by a pervasive and persistent distrust and suspicion of others. They are hypersensitive in general with others and are difficult to be in a relationship with since they are suspicious and controlling and can be obsessive. They may be into conspiracy theories and can get angry if they are challenged. They are difficult to get along with and have difficulty making close friends. Their paranoia and fear are not matched by reality.

If a mood disorder is also associated, then the likelihood is much higher that the patient has bipolar disorder rather than unipolar disorder. The patient may even have schizoaffective disorder or even paranoid schizophrenia, though some people have the personality type but no treatable neurochemical imbalances that can be fixed with the proper psychotropic medications. Thankfully that is rare.

The reality is that most of these patients benefit from psychotropic medications at some level, since with a personality that is exaggerated and extreme there is likely a coexisting mood disorder that is significant, whether it is unipolar or bipolar, and thankfully we have the means to treat either or both together and allow our patients to live their lives to the fullest.

As I have repeatedly mentioned, medications can mellow out the personality and thus make it easier to be around the person. The majority of these patients are men, and they are usually more of a harm to themselves than they are to others, who feel they are just strange and a bit "off."

The schizoid personality disorder is characterized by a tendency to maintain physical and emotional distance from others, avoiding encounters and interactions. They are frequently loners because of the discomfort they feel around others. Others also may feel uncomfortable around them since they seem so weird and strange. They can't relax around other people and appear emotionally flat, cold, and distant. These patients are usually male and, more often than not, have an underlying mood disorder that coexists.

They are more likely unipolar than bipolar. They may have Bipolar I Disorder or other lesser versions, sometimes manic or hypomanic and more often depressed, as well as a more severe form such as Schizoaffective Disorder or even Schizophrenia. Medications usually help to mellow out the personality, though the underlying characteristics are very difficult to change, even with therapy.

The schizotypal personality disorder characteristics are even more bizarre in certain ways. They are very socially awkward and very quirky in their mannerisms and behaviors. They have a deeply rooted sense of inadequacy and social impotence. They tend to isolate because of their awkwardness and have difficulty making close friends or getting along with their family and friends. They may be drawn to strange beliefs and superstitions and may have magical thinking. They may dress awkwardly and stand out, which is really not what they want. This is more likely among men than women. They more often than not have one or more underlying mood disorders that can be treated and thus reduce the impact of the personality on themselves and on others.

They are more likely bipolar than unipolar, and may have coexisting Bipolar I Disorder or a lesser version, along with schizoaffective disorder or even schizophrenia. As is the case with all personality disorders, it is very difficult to change the core personality traits of a person no matter what therapy is applied, though some types are better than others for these patients. People typically don't change unless they want to, and even if they want to, that is still difficult to accomplish. However, these patients can also be very interesting to work with and exciting to treat if you're into it like I am.

IV: Antisocial Personality Disorder (ASPD) The Most Dangerous Types

Antisocial Personality Disorder is the last group that I will discuss. They are also the most dangerous and most disturbing ones, the sociopaths and psychopaths. They are the most dysfunctional and can cause immense damage to the lives of others. These are the thugs and common criminals. They are the wrong crowd to hang out with. If their morals and values declined to the point of not having empathy and feelings for others and caring for others when appropriate, then this leads to full-blown sociopathy, which is just one step away from psychopathy.

Sociopaths and psychopaths are very disturbed individuals that have no remorse or empathy for their victims. They thrive on power and control. They are very self-centered, like narcissists, and focus only on their twisted needs and desires. They don't care about the suffering of others but rather actually enjoy it. They lack any type of moral compass, lack values, and ultimately have no soul.

When evil combines with these more dangerous personality disorders, the consequences can be severe. It can even be a matter of life or death. Treating underlying mood disorders in this group only does so much. Psychotropic medications can help the mood, but they do not restore ethics, values, and morality. Their best chance to change is a true spiritual conversion.

Psychopathic Personality Disorder is the most extreme and severe, such as murderers, rapists, and others that are prone to violence and mayhem. They thrive on power and control over others. The sociopaths, though, can be dangerous in their own right in many ways. I strongly refer you to an amazing book, *The Sociopath Next Door* by Dr. Martha Stout, PhD, a psychologist that specializes in treating victims of sociopaths. I agree with her advice to stay away from these people as much as possible. Get away and don't look back. At least have only the minimal contact needed. Be careful and don't be fooled. Assume that they won't change, while holding on to the slim hope that they eventually will.

12) High Achievers

There are many with bipolar disorder who are extremely accomplished and successful. They can be excellent students and are often brilliant. Some of them are even geniuses. They can be very driven, and it can be difficult to outwork them since they are willing to put in whatever hours and do whatever is needed to get the job done. Having this disorder can, in a way, be a gift as long as the negative parts are controlled.

Bipolar patients tend to have higher intelligence than their unipolar counterparts, though that really depends on the person. They may be brimming with confidence but can tend to have a lack of judgment and insight. They didn't like to take responsibility for their actions and often blamed others and may even play the victim role.

When they are manic or hypomanic, their minds are racing, and they get a lot done since they're workaholics and they don't need much sleep, or they don't think they do. Ultimately, however, this state can't last forever, and then they may crash into depression. During this state also, the thinking may not be rational. It's very difficult to rationalize with an irrational mind and person.

There are many wealthy people and celebrities that are bipolar, and part of the reason they got to where they did is partially because of their bipolarity since some of the features can actually be an asset. Great inventions and works of art, music, writing, etc., are sometimes accomplished while the patient is in a manic state, when the person feels more creative and is able to put in long hours. A big problem with treating this is that many patients who are in that state do not want me to take their edge away by tuning them down with mood stabilizers, so they are notoriously noncompliant. When they are feeling good and getting a lot done, it's quite difficult to talk them into giving that up. Even if they know that it will not last, they may want to ride that wave as long as they can until it crashes. Some have grandiose thinking and feelings of special powers and insight. The problem, though, can be that they have very little insight into themselves and don't really understand what other people see or think about them, since they are in the "zone" and don't want to be interrupted or distracted in any way.

Hypomania is what I refer to as "mania lite" since it has a lighter effect than mania does. It is a more functional state since there is less or none of the irrationality, paranoia, intense fears, and fear of the manic state. They can be very successful, and it can be difficult to outwork them since they are very driven people. The mood, however, is more elevated than a normal individual, so it is still difficult to talk them into changing that state of being.

Hypomania is a state of being in-between mania and euthymia (euthymia being the person's "normal" mood). Hypomanics usually sleep better than manic patients, but they also usually have some issue with their sleep. However, they also don't need as much sleep as the average person or one with unipolar depression. People who have experienced this shifting of mood want to stay in the hypomanic state, but unfortunately the positive aspect doesn't last since the person may then shift into either mania or a potentially deep depression.

The riskiest is the manic state, but also risky is severe depression when one drops into the lower pole, which in bipolar disorder is usually much more common than the manic or hypomanic states. After the person is steeped into deep depression, they then long to feel how they felt when they were at their "best," which is actually not really their best and healthiest. These are especially high-risk times for suicidal thinking and behaviors, so it is important that this is adequately screened for.

They are usually more open to being treated when they are depressed rather than when they are hypomanic and feeling quite well and don't see the need to change or have the desire to do so. Patients who are trapped in a deep depression typically want to get out of it, though there are some who are resistant to treatment in a medical way since they do not see this problem as medical but only as psychological or situational. In reality it is typically a combination of all these together. Some people in actuality feel comfortable being depressed, as strange as that sounds. They may even consider it "normal" for them. My job is to get them out of their comfort zone and accept a healthy treatment plan in order to get them to a healthier "new normal."

As I said, people are more likely to accept help when they are depressed, and it is the practitioner's job to convince them to follow through with our medical advice. We need to get good and comfortable with convincing people who need help to follow through with our recommendations. Some patients stay at the mania and hypomania level and don't get depressed, which is fortunate for them as long as they realize they still should treat the upper pole in order to tune the brain down to normal. Patients who are trapped in depression more often than not want to get out of it, though there are some who are resistant to being treated and don't believe in the psychotropic medication approach. Some people feel comfortable wallowing in their misery and, in a strange sense, feel comfortable being depressed because it is what they know. They may even feel that suffering is noble. In this case I try to convince them otherwise since there is no reason that someone should suffer needlessly.

Bipolar patients are very sensitive to antidepressants and often need lower doses than their unipolar counterparts. It's also important to use adequate mood stabilizers to prevent antidepressants from destabilizing the mood by bringing on hypomania and especially mania. Most patients, though, need both classes in order to achieve full remission. Mood stabilizers also have the advantage of having antidepressant actions so that they treat both poles of the disorder, though the addition of antidepressants is almost always warranted.

Psychotherapy can also be helpful, as well as relaxation techniques and a spiritual connection. Whichever stage the bipolar person is at, it is important to treat them correctly in order to obtain the most complete stability and optimal functionality of that person. Even though they are often brilliant, successful, and admired, in order for them to continue that way, it is important to have the mood stabilized when needed in order for that person to be his or her best, most in control, and happy in their lives.

13) Psychosomatic Complaints

Mind-body disorders are so common, and the odds are more likely that those who suffer with the emotional and physical changes have unipolar disorder rather than bipolar disorder since it just happens more frequently.

However, what is discounted is how common bipolar disorder really is, since it is so underrecognized and more often than not misdiagnosed. The reality for many, though, is that they have a combination of both, which can present in such a more subtle fashion than the obvious mania and irrationality that goes along with Bipolar I Disorder. Even though psychosomatic symptoms occur in both, the presentation can be more dramatic and intensified in the bipolar patients.

The most common psychosomatic symptoms are diverse and can include headaches; neck, shoulder, and upper back pain; TMJ/jaw pain caused by nighttime teeth grinding; Irritable Bowel Syndrome (IBS); fibromyalgia; dysmenorrhea (painful menstruation); chronic recurring pain in any area of the body; acute or chronic fatigue; skin conditions; neurological symptoms; and recurring infections. These symptoms can manifest in a variety of ways.

They may be treatment-resistant in some cases, since medications can really only do so much and only change what they can. It's also important to realize that if the wrong psychotropic medications are given to patients with the wrong diagnosis, then of course this would be problematic.

Bipolar patients may need higher doses of pain pills, antianxiety agents, sleeping pills, and other "band-aid" solutions that treat only the symptoms but ignore the underlying true cause. Not only do bipolar patients need more symptomatic treatments, but they also need higher than normal doses of the mood stabilizers, while at the same time often needing lower than average doses of antidepressants, since they often get quick results even at the lowest doses.

The two usual chemicals that are imbalanced in more severe psychosomatic cases are norepinephrine and GABA, though serotonin and dopamine may also be involved. An SNRI-GABAergic combination is the "Dynamic Duo" in the psychosomatic realm. Whether the patient is unipolar or bipolar norepinephrine and GABA are important chemicals to account for and take seriously, not just serotonin and dopamine.

I usually think of norepinephrine first and then GABA second for unipolar patients and those on the lower bipolar spectrum, while I think of GABA first for bipolar patients who have psychosomatic issues (along with dopamine, of course), and then follow up with a norepinephrine agent when appropriate. Some doctors feel that SNRIs should be totally avoided if the patient has bipolar disorder. This may be the case with the higher grade Bipolar I or even possibly Bipolar II, but that rule is often not the case. If one is chosen for the right patient, then the results can be quite spectacular while being well-tolerated at the same time.

Not only are medications important, but it's also important to exercise regularly, practice relaxation techniques, and live a healthy lifestyle. These healthy habits go a long way towards becoming fully better. However difficult it is to treat, and no matter whether it is related more to bipolar, unipolar or somewhere in-between, it is important to be treated most optimally using whatever works by utilizing the best treatment strategies. Whatever we need to do to help these patients is worth the effort, and thankfully that reality is achievable the vast majority of the time.

14) Hospitalization

It is certainly the case that many unipolar patients end up in the hospital if they are morbidly depressed, in a highly manic state, suicidal, or if they are noncompliant with treatment. However, hospitalization definitely increases the potential that the patient is really in the bipolar spectrum rather than the unipolar spectrum. The criteria for hospitalization are when the person is a danger to himself or herself or is a danger to others. Otherwise, in my opinion, it is advisable that the person be treated in an outpatient setting, since the care is more individualized and the setting is more comfortable. They still need to be closely observed, though, hopefully with the involvement of people they are close to, such as family and friends.

In an inpatient setting, patients have very little contact with the psychiatrist and basically are being protected from themselves by being closely monitored and by ensuring that they take their medications properly. It is usually not at all a pleasant environment, and the patient is often surrounded by people who are way worse, which can be a bit scary to be around, and they can become very homesick at that point. There is a little group counseling, mostly with group sessions, but basically it is a waste of time and money if one is not acutely ill.

If medications need to be monitored closely, then that is another good reason for inpatient observation, otherwise, most patients can be treated in an outpatient setting safely and effectively. Since bipolar disorder presents in a more dramatic fashion, suicidal ideation and planning certainly are as dramatic and dangerous as they get. The number one priority should be resolution of suicidal ideation, whether it be a "cry for attention and help" or a true plan of action.

It is important, whether in an inpatient setting or, much more likely, an outpatient setting, that the person is treated in the most complete and effective way. In an inpatient setting the treatment is more aggressive than it would be in an outpatient setting due to close monitoring in order to be able to discharge the patient as quickly and as safely as possible. Another reason that they titrate quickly to a higher dose of one or more mood stabilizers is to sedate the person so that he or she is more easily controllable by the staff to make their jobs easier.

15) Suicidality

Even though suicidal thinking can occur in both unipolar and bipolar disorders, this is a definite hint that we need to at least look in the bipolar direction when assessing the person. The higher the level and severity of the bipolar patient, the more likely suicidal thinking and suicidality, though even lower grades of bipolar and unipolar disorders have a common factor of suicidal thinking for some. The risk of completing suicide is higher in the bipolar than the unipolar patients.

Many have what I refer to as "passive" suicidal thinking. They may tell us that if they don't wake up tomorrow, they are okay with that, or have a desire to escape and get away from the situation, though most of them say they wouldn't actually follow through with it. We need to appreciate, however, that a significant number of people are completing the act, so we have to be sensitive to this in order to prevent them from following through with the threat. It's a great idea to make a verbal contract with these patients. I have them promise me that they will not act on the ideation. I assure them that they will feel much better, but I just need time in order to get the treatment just so. It has been shown that verbal contracts like this are very effective.

I also make it clear that if they are thinking about following through with the ideation, they can contact me or another person that they can get in touch with quickly. When our clients know that we and others care about them, then they have more hope that there is a light at the end of the tunnel and that they are really going to get better.

Psychotropic medications are most definitely the "gold standard" when it comes to treatment at whichever level the person is at until the patient is a fully functional person who loves life and doesn't want it to end. There is a misconception and a myth that antidepressants increase the risk of suicide. This is simply not the case, no matter if it's a child, an adolescent, a young adult, or later. It has been believed that it especially increases the risk in teenagers and young adults.

This misperception by the government occurred, in my opinion, when they studied this issue. They lumped all patients together and didn't distinguish which were the unipolar patients and which were the bipolar patients. Since unipolar disorder is more common, the vast majority of patients who need antidepressants improve dramatically. If they work very well quickly but then become hypomanic or manic, it can be decided whether to add a mood stabilizer, temporarily stop the antidepressant, or both. This uncovers the need for treatment of the upper pole with the correct medication class. Since the response to medications is so quick, we can make quick decisions when it comes to what to add, what to delete, and how to augment properly.

The risk of suicide increases if the patient is diagnosed with MDD but actually has bipolar disorder. In these cases, if an antidepressant can switch the patient from depression into mania, then there is the risk that the person is energized and irrational. Even though the risk is still low, it is crucial then to stop the offending agent and quickly change the treatment course.

This misperception of the supposed danger of antidepressants has unfortunately led to a profound lack of treatment that is needed. Some patients stopped taking them, some parents were afraid to treat their children, and some people decided against taking them at all.

When the FDA posted these warnings years ago, I was very upset when I read an article about it in our local newspaper. I wanted to warn everyone that I could at the time as to what the impact would be. I wrote a lengthy editorial about this and sent it to the local newspaper, but it never got published. Unfortunately, this action has led to many unnecessary deaths. Until that time suicide rates had been decreasing with the modern antidepressants, starting with Prozac (fluoxetine). Since then, as I had warned, suicide rates have increased dramatically. My best advice is to never take medical advice from the government, which is just like getting medical advice from attorneys, which I do not recommend.

If we are aware of bipolar disorder then we, of course, are more cautious when it comes to treatment. We realize that if the patient is more unstable, then a mood stabilizer would be the best next choice, possibly followed by an antidepressant, a second mood stabilizer, or both. The key is to treat the most acute problem first and then do the rest in order of importance. Preventing suicide is obviously our number one priority with patients, and once you get past that, the rest is easier and safer.

Summary

There are a lot of clues along the way when it comes to solving the puzzle of whether the patient is bipolar or not. We need to look at the whole history, analyzing each minor piece of the puzzle along the way. We need to look at changes over time by documenting the person's life from start to the current state, focusing on times when instability occurred and changed the person for the worse or better. We need to look at cyclical changes over the years, whether high or low, noting each detail about what we uncover.

I also look strongly at family history, since this can give a lot of clues that are helpful while assessing the patient. I take a full history of antidepressants tried as well as any other medications attempted and hone in on the details of each medication experience, whether good, bad, or indifferent. If antidepressants either don't work or work too quickly and destabilize a patient, then this is very helpful in order to diagnose what is really going on. In that case mood stabilizers can be quickly added, usually without the need to withdraw the helpful antidepressants that may seem too helpful too quickly. Since both classes of medications, antidepressants and mood stabilizers, work so quickly and effectively, we can make quick decisions regarding the titration of each medication.

I also look at the severity of symptoms and the response of them to treatment. If symptoms are more severe and more resistant to antidepressant treatment, then this is a hint that the patient is on the bipolar end of the mood spectrum. If the patient needs high doses of pain medications, muscle relaxants, benzodiazepines/minor tranquilizers, sleeping pills, or whichever symptomatic treatment, then this is a hint that we need to strongly consider bipolar instead of a unipolar problem.

If the patient has mood swings and erratic behavior, then bipolar should definitely be considered. When insomnia is a significant factor in the mood disorder, then it is more likely that the patient tilts in the bipolar direction, especially if the brain has difficulty turning off even with treatment. If antidepressants worsen mood, then this is another clue that the wrong pole is being addressed.

At that point we can shift our treatment course in the right direction and make the necessary adjustments in order to create the perfect recipe for success. We need to keep an open mind when we are evaluating patients to look for subtle presentations that are meaningful if we know what we are looking for and then what to do with that crucial information. Bipolar disorder is one of my favorite diagnoses to treat, since I enjoy the challenge it presents and since the results are so dramatic and life-altering for our patients as well as all the others in their lives. I have the pleasure of being able to witness these life-changing treatments firsthand so often, and it is exciting to see what a dramatic impact proper treatment makes.

Going back to that Seroquel (quetiapine) and Seroquel XR (quetiapine ER) speaker training conference, I was hearing that 10% of bipolar disorder was type I, 20% is bipolar II, and

70% is bipolar disorder not otherwise specified (NOS), which means that 70% of bipolar disorder is from the spectrum, such as bipolar 3 to bipolar 6 or more. The presentations may not be as obvious as four days of hypomania needed for the Bipolar 2 diagnosis, which presents as elevated mood and a decreased need for sleep, without irrational thinking or behaviors. However, this state of being doesn't last, and eventually the person can swing to the upper or lower pole or develop a mixed state, meaning both at the same time.

How about those patients that have one to three days of hypomania, thus not falling within the criteria of four days to meet the criteria for Bipolar 2 Disorder? The point I'm trying to make here is that there is so much variability and individuality when it comes to the variety of subtle presentations. This is why I like the term bipolar spectrum disorder, since so many patients fall within the spectrum.

When the patient is in a hypomanic state, though, with an elevated mood, a decreased need for sleep, and plenty of creativity and ideas, that person may feel at the peak of his or her performance, so why change, right? It can be difficult to advise and convince them otherwise.

Mood stabilizers are an important part of the equation, which I consider to be the atypical antipsychotics, the GABAergic medications, and the traditional mood stabilizers lithium carbonate and Depakote. I only prescribe one medication at a time, though we can still be as aggressive regarding treatment as we need to be. I often mix mood stabilizers together, as I do with antidepressants, and then attempt to create the perfect cocktail. Two to three medications are the usual minimum amount needed, with more than three likely for more complex patients like the higher-grade bipolar patients.

Treating bipolar disorder in the most complete and effective way takes a lot of practice and a good feel for it in order to optimize the positive effects while minimizing the negative aspects of psychotropic medications, mainly the antidepressants and mood stabilizers. It takes good instincts for what each person needs as an individual in order to treat it in the best preventative and holistic way.

Understanding that the reason it takes 3 to 4 doctors and 7 to 10 years to properly diagnose bipolar disorder is that it is not being recognized adequately for what it really is, which includes primary care providers such as family physicians, internists, and pediatricians, as well as physician assistants, nurse practitioners, and psychiatrists. If doctors can get on board and see how commonly it presents and how easy it is to treat, then this would improve the quality of life of patients who so desperately need this type of help. The more we learn to treat each individual, the better it is for us, our patients, and society as a whole.

It is vital to treat the mind and body completely and at the same time by doing whatever is needed neurochemically, hormonally, emotionally, physically, and spiritually in order to create the ultimate mind-body connection with peace and harmony from within.

SECRET #3

Recognizing the Importance of Getting Patients to Achieve Full Remission

SECRET #3

Recognizing the Importance of Getting Patients to Achieve Full Remission

Full and complete remission is quite simply the "gold standard" of successful treatment for every individual patient we see. This is the state of being when the person is fully well, either back to their old self or even better than that. When we take a full history about the premorbid condition of the patient to find out when things started to go wrong, this is the place that we need to get them back to, using whichever tools we have in the tool chest in order to make that happen.

When a patient suffers with emotional and physical ailments, remission is the state of no longer experiencing significant clinical symptoms with regard to mood and emotions, as well as somatic/physical symptoms. Remission is, simply put, the indicator of complete wellness, and it is the goal for every patient to achieve.

In order to better explain remission in a more exact way, there are many different rating scales that patients can fill out and that clinicians can use to evaluate and score the severity of the condition. In my first book I mentioned the HAM-D when I discussed the topic of remission. The 17-item Hamilton Rating Scale for Depression (HAM-D17) has been used for four decades as the "gold standard" instrument to assess the severity of depression and response to therapy in clinical research. A score of 0–7 indicates a normal state, 8 to 13 mild depression, 14 to 18 moderate depression, 19 to 22 severe depression, and 23 or more indicating very severe depression. The higher the score, the worse the depression, and as is the case in golf, the lower the score, the better.

It is important to understand the terms "response" and "remission" in order to prevent recurrence and relapse. A response indicates an "adequate" treatment outcome of a medication trial in order for a medication to be approved by the FDA. Using the HAM-D, if a medication trial produces a 50% improvement of the score, that is considered a response. For example, if the patient starts off with a score of 30, which indicates a significantly severe depression, and if after a medication trial the score comes down to 15, that is a 50% improvement from baseline and thus considered to be an adequate response to the medication. At first glance this looks great since the patient goes from very severe depression to the mild to moderate range, but that is still not good enough.

The goal is to get to 7 or less on the scale, which indicates normal mood without any significant depression. However, the real goal is to get to zero, or at least as close as we can realistically get. That means in this case that we still have more than 50% of the way to go after the previous intervention in order to achieve the ultimate goal of full and complete remission. It is widely understood that the importance of achieving full remission is because this minimizes the risk of recurrence and relapse. If the patient is stuck in the state of response, then we will not reach the ultimate goal that we need to achieve, and that is unacceptable. We must do much better than that for our patients if we really want to get them completely well now and over the long term.

The goal of remission is not only to prevent recurrence and relapse, but remission also means that the patient is able to achieve optimal social and occupational functioning. When the person is in response, there still may be significant residual psychological and physical problems that stand in the way of patients feeling their best. Since I don't use rating scales in my practice, I get a detailed history and take stock of all of the symptoms that are working against the patient, and each visit I try to make progress resolving each of these symptoms as we work toward getting the patient closer to full remission by the next visit. If we're not there yet, then the next visit I do the same until we have reached our goal.

It is important to document the symptoms and progress clearly in the chart so that the notes are easy to follow so that we can clearly see that we are working towards achieving our goals. Most certainly in my case, as well for many doctors, it is best to not always rely on handwritten notes but rather on dictation or digital notes. Anyone who has seen my handwritten notes understands this.

The symptoms I look for include psychological and emotional as well as physical symptoms that relate to the mood and the physical body at the same time. I keep track of each visit as to how much closer we are to our goal, and then I do whatever is needed in order to achieve the ultimate prize.

In addition to a full assessment of symptoms, we also need to understand the premorbid condition of the patient in order to figure out whether we are making adequate progress or not towards the goal of complete remission. Some patients definitely know the times of their lives when they felt and functioned at their best, with the most common answers being elementary school/early childhood and early to mid 20s, since these years tend to be more carefree, when life is less complex and stressful and more about just having fun as well as getting a proper education or learning a trade in order to achieve a happy and prosperous life. For some people the optimal time is after having kids and raising them. I try to figure out whichever time or times that were the very best for each individual, and then I try my best to do everything I can to get that person back to that happiest place, and sometimes even better.

However, other patients have horrific backgrounds and life experiences and have gone through a lot of trauma, so they don't really know what it feels like to live a happy and carefree life. For these patients our goal is to help them to see what "normal" feels like for the first time in their lives in whatever way we can. If we continue to take detailed notes and track every emotional and physical symptom visit by visit (or better yet, the lack of them), we will be able to tell when we have gone as far as we can and then continue to work on keeping them there. We should never be satisfied until the patient is fully well, which is when full and complete remission is achieved and maintained over time.

I will now provide you in this section with a list of symptoms that I focus on when assessing patients both emotionally and physically. I encourage every new patient to call me after one week of our first visit to update me. (No, I don't charge for these phone calls in-between visits. I'm not an attorney.) During these calls I can tweak the medication to see the results firsthand prior to the follow-up visit in the following week or two. I can tell within that first week if I gave the person the right medication or not. If not, I can quickly change course since it's so important to get the first piece right. This also shows patients that I care, which I most certainly do.

I then continue to encourage patients to update me by phone and/or email in-between visits if things are not going as I hoped. Titration as well as augmentation can be done during these relatively brief phone calls or emails. A lot of progress can be accomplished if we work quickly and efficiently and continue to have good communication. Being available also adds a personal touch and shows people that I truly care about them and their mental and physical health. Patients are typically not used to this type of personalized care and customer service and are pleasantly surprised since it is difficult to find in this profession.

I continue to tweak the medications until I see the most satisfactory results, which means the resolution of all the negative symptoms and optimization of mood. Then we continue longer-term follow-up to make sure that the state of remission is maintained over time to both of our satisfaction.

Fatigue

This is a very common symptom and complaint among patients. Even though fatigue is commonly caused by neurochemical imbalances, there are other potential reasons we need to explore. Fatigue can most certainly affect the quality and efficiency of the day in some fashion. It is important to rule out potential medical problems, which can be worked up, explored, and exposed. This helps to clarify the direction of treatment. We may need to address it in a combination of ways. Fatigue can also be a byproduct of treatment with antidepressants and mood stabilizers, but whatever the reason for the fatigue, it is important to resolve this if one hopes to achieve full remission.

When it comes to the antidepressant classes, fatigue is more common with SSRIs than SNRIs and is even less common with Wellbutrin. We need to assess whether the positive benefits outweigh the fatigue that we can deal with in other ways and whether there is a better medication to try instead. Once we find the best first antidepressant fit, if fatigue is present, then we can address it in other ways. It's important to get the first antidepressant just right, since it's easier to build upon a good foundation.

The most common augmentation strategy that I employ to address fatigue is the addition of Wellbutrin XL, since this dopaminergic kick can help to offset the potentially sedating effects of balancing serotonin or even norepinephrine with an SNRI or with GABAergic medications. Wellbutrin also helps to boost dopamine and norepinephrine when given with a dopamine antagonist. This suppresses dopamine and serotonin when that type of balance is needed. Wellbutrin can have a symbiotic effect by boosting dopamine when needed while the atypical antipsychotic slows it down when needed, which I refer to as balancing dopamine 24/7.

A newer name-brand bupropion XL to compete with Wellbutrin XL is Aplenzin, which is a high-quality version and sometimes a little better and better tolerated than the generic version. An advantage that Aplenzin has is that the company provides samples so that we can actually try it and compare it side-by-side to Wellbutrin XL to see if it is worth switching or not. However, it is difficult to critique the generic version, since I have had decades of excellent experiences with it.

The newest antidepressant on the market is formatted as a very powerful and effective agent for those who have treatment-resistant depression. I reach for these samples if Wellbutrin XL doesn't work as I would expect it to or if it works but then "poops out." It is a combination of Wellbutrin SR, which, as we know boosts dopamine as well as norepinephrine, along with dextromethorphan, which boosts glutamate, and it indirectly also modulates and boosts serotonin a bit as well as norepinephrine a bit more. If I believe that the patient is within the unipolar spectrum rather than the bipolar spectrum, I would try this first before considering an atypical antipsychotic.

Other augmenting choices include Provigil (modafinil), Nuvigil (armodafinil), Sunosi (solriamfetol), Deplin (L-methylfolate), and/or a stimulant. If sedation is a significant factor with an SSRI or an SNRI, there needs to be at least significant progress in order to keep it and then augment with Wellbutrin XL. Otherwise, it is possible that serotonin and/or norepinephrine are not significant issues, and if this is the case, it is reasonable to use Wellbutrin XL as the first-line antidepressant. However, the odds are that it is more likely beneficial as an augmenting agent. Adding Wellbutrin to other antidepressants not only can help energy but also overall mood at the same time, which is why augmentation should be the rule for most patients, with monotherapy being the exception.

When I hear of patients' symptoms such as not only fatigue but also apathy, poor motivation and drive, isolating and not wanting to engage with others, poor sex drive and functioning, poor focus and concentration, poor memory, and difficulty with functioning in general throughout the day, as well as overall lack of joy and happiness, I think of dopamine first, which is why I refer to dopamine as the "pleasure chemical."

If fatigue is a significant problem, then there are other possible reasons to explore rather than just neurochemical ones. We need to do a full lab assessment to explore medical factors that can cause fatigue, such as anemia, hypothyroidism, vitamin deficiency, or other etiologies. I also focus on healthy lifestyle habits such as a well-balanced diet and a regular cardiovascular exercise program. The key is the intensity and consistency of the exercise regimen. Once potential medical, psychological, and lifestyle reasons have been ruled out, then we can focus our attention on the neurochemical realm for answers. We need to pay attention to which antidepressant leads to the best efficacy and the fewest side effects, such as fatigue and others.

We also need to realize that mood stabilizers are not only often the cause of improved efficacy but also potentially may be causing fatigue as a side effect. If this is the case, though, then we may need to switch to a different one that won't be sedating. However, as is the case with antidepressants, it may take trying different mood stabilizers until we get the best results with the least fatigue and other side effects. However, if fatigue is still a factor regardless of our choice, then thankfully, we have very good tools available that can help us resolve this problem.

The reality is that a cocktail of medications like The Corona Cocktails, which is based on the rational polypharmaceutical approach, which is based on trial-and-error, is the best approach to address imbalanced neurochemicals. We won't be able to achieve full remission if fatigue persists. It needs to be addressed in safe and effective ways. If it is not addressed properly, then fatigue can hold people back from getting back to their old selves or feeling even better than that emotionally and physically.

Insomnia, Bipolar Disorder, and Addiction

This is another common symptom that will occur due to an underlying mood disorder. It can also be a potential side effect from psychotropics as well as other medications. If it is not resolved, it can definitely keep people from feeling their best. Insomnia is now considered a psychiatric "vital sign" that we need to track along the way since it is so important that it is addressed and appropriately resolved. Insomnia is a common condition related to different disorders such as depression, anxiety disorders, bipolar disorders, and others.

Depressive patients often have early-morning awakenings, going to sleep okay but waking up in the 2–4 a.m. range and having difficulty getting back to sleep. Anxious patients may have more difficulty getting to sleep than staying asleep, though both types of patients can have both. Bipolar patients have more difficulty getting to sleep and staying asleep, since the mind is racing and it can be difficult to settle it down, thus causing difficulty sleeping throughout the night.

Bipolar patients have a decreased need to sleep and may function fine the next day, whereas depressed and anxious patients are more likely to suffer the consequence of fatigue the next day. A decreased need for sleep is a significant symptom that points clearly towards the bipolar spectrum.

Insomnia may also be a consequence of treatment with antidepressants or even mood stabilizers, so we need to assess whether a medication that does so can be switched to a different one that doesn't cause the side effect, or if the results are very good, we can then deal with the side effect in other ways. We need to make sure that each medication we choose has the best efficacy and side effect profile, and this may take some trial-and-error in order to figure this out.

It's also possible that a medication that leads to insomnia is actually uncovering another underlying mood disorder that is hiding under the surface that wasn't previously appreciated. In these cases, we may need to alter our approach in order to treat these diagnoses until all of the symptoms are adequately resolved, which is necessary in order to achieve remission.

It is important to get a complete history of the patient's sleep pattern in order to see when it was not an issue and when that changed and why. It could have started with situational stressors or may have started with the onset of unipolar or bipolar disorder. It may very well be a combination of factors, such as sleep apnea or other underlying medical factors, such as diabetes and many others, that needs to be evaluated and addressed.

When it comes to the bedtime hours, this is when things slow down and the mind has time to think. Worry and obsess about the past, and worry about the next day and beyond. A person is most vulnerable during the hours that are set aside for sleep, when it is dark and quiet and there is nothing else going on.

If a medication is causing insomnia or uncovering another mood disorder, then it depends if it is worth keeping it and then dealing with the insomnia or switching to a potentially better choice that may not cause this side effect. We also need to keep in mind that other factors can lead to insomnia, such as excessive use of caffeine, nicotine, alcohol, or street drugs. Methamphetamines are the most dangerous class when it comes to bipolar patients, which is like pouring gasoline on a fire. If an antidepressant or an illicit substance uncovers bipolar traits that were not previously recognized, then it may just be easiest if the patient is stable or not too unstable to add a mood stabilizer, such as an atypical antipsychotic, a GABAergic medication, a "classic" mood stabilizer like lithium carbonate or Depakote, or a combination thereof.

The Gold Standard for Sleep

Seroquel (quetiapine) is the gold standard to address insomnia, though for some it is a bit too potent and too sedating the next day. Many of the other atypicals are also excellent for sleep quality, such as Risperdal (risperidone), Zyprexa (olanzapine), Saphris (asenapine), Invega (paliperidone), Latuda, Caplyta (lumateperone), Lybalvi (olanzapine and samidorphan), and Fanapt (iloperidone). The GABAergic medications, such as Depakote, Topamax (topiramate), gabapentin, Trileptal (oxcarbazepine), and others, may also help with sleep. Trazodone is one of the most common choices, with the advantage of not being a controlled substance. Remeron (mirtazapine), low-dose tricyclic antidepressants such as doxepin and others, alpha blockers, and other medication choices are available.

There are the tranquilizing sleeping pills that have been around for a long time, which are Ambien (zolpidem) and Lunesta (eszopiclone). The newest is Quviviq, one of three dual orexin receptor antagonists along with Belsomra and Dayvigo. There are also benzodiazepines such as Xanax (alprazolam), Klonopin (clonazepam), Ativan (lorazepam), Valium (diazepam), and others, though those are best reserved for anxiety attacks rather than for sleep. There are many over-the-counter products that often contain Benadryl or other antihistamines.

There are also herbal remedies that work for some, such as melatonin, kava kava, GABA supplements, tryptophan, magnesium, and many other herbal choices. I try to keep the benzodiazepines and sleeping pills as "last-line," since other more first-line and preventative choices that I just mentioned not only improve the sleep quality but also may improve the mood at the same time. If we do not optimally treat the underlying mood disorder that causes the insomnia and just cover it up with a "band-aid," then they will not be feeling the best that they can.

I prefer to maximize the preventative and nonaddictive medications such as antidepressants and mood stabilizers and then minimize the symptomatic medications needed with potentially addictive products that also may cause side effects and increase the risk of addiction and dependence if one is prone to it. There are also concerns about cognitive side effects and even early dementia with the use of too many tranquilizers over time. If the results are good, then it is reasonable to just treat in a preventative way by maximizing the nonaddictive preventative medications.

Sometimes though the "band-aids" are needed for people to get relief from insomnia, since if we do not resolve this issue, then this will hold back the patient from achieving full remission. Medications are not the only option to help with sleep, since relaxation techniques such as proper breathing, mindfulness, yoga, meditation, contemplative prayer, and a regular cardiovascular exercise program, as well as other modalities, can help. It's so important to get the rest that is needed in order to be able to function at our best. Sleep optimization is huge, so we need to learn to best treat it in a healthy and preventative way.

The more difficulty the patient has with sleep, the more likely the patient is bipolar instead of unipolar. The higher the doses of medications needed that help with sleep and relaxation, as well as when more medications are needed to resolve this, then we need to be thinking in a bipolar direction of the spectrum.

In these cases, we need to address any addiction issues and try to resolve those while at the same time focusing on adequate mood stabilization. In order to get the most proper diagnosis, there are some simple screening questions we can ask in order to differentiate whether the insomnia is from anxiety or depressive episodes.

In order to tease out hypomania or mania, I typically first inquire what is the longest period of time they can recall going without sleep or with decreased sleep. I then clarify if he or she wanted to sleep and couldn't fall asleep or if they didn't want to sleep because they felt they didn't need to sleep. I then ask if, after the decreased sleep or a few nights without sleep, they were tired and felt that they wanted to sleep. If they were tired after not sleeping well for a few days, then I am less suspicious of a bipolar diathesis.

If they continued to have lots of energy and didn't feel tired, then I hone in on the bipolar criteria. For hypomania (mania-lite, a milder, more rational, and more functional version), they need at least four days of decreased/no sleep, though between two and three days is significant in my opinion. Even one day or less may be an important sign that we need to recognize that and keep an open mind about the extremely subtle bipolar presentations.

For mania they need at least one week of decreased/no sleep or required hospitalization. I also assess whether mood lability is a factor. If moods last minutes to hours, then this could just be due to the patient's disordered personality, such as a borderline personality disorder presentation. If the mood swings, though, occur over hours to days, then this may be more of a bipolar type of mood lability. We can hone in on the specific periods of time and specific symptoms during those episodes, such as need for sleep, irrational thinking, irrational behaviors, paranoia and risk-taking activities and behaviors.

Addiction needs to be screened for, and this issue needs to be adequately dealt with in order for the patient to move hopefully toward the life of sobriety. By taking a good history and following our patients closely, we can resolve the problem of insomnia in whichever way we need to. Sleep is just that important. If insomnia is properly dealt with, it is much more likely that full remission will be achieved and will persist over time.

Psychosomatic Complaints

Somatic symptoms are often overlooked as being related to mood and emotion. Most psychiatrists understand emotion and mood but often don't understand the link to the physical body. There are formal psychiatric diagnoses in the DSM-5 that include somatic components, but that is not emphasized in psychiatry, so it is not surprising that many psychiatrists don't understand and appreciate the importance of the mind-body connection.

What is surprising is that even after certain somatic disorders have been included in the DSM-5, and even after psychotropic medications have come out that address physical and not just emotional symptoms, there is still this profound lack of recognition of the intimate relations between physical and mental health. Otherwise, their patients will never get completely better.

I won't let primary care doctors or mid-level practitioners such as PAs and NPs off the hook though, because they also unfortunately miss this important link. Our training in primary care focused on the physical body. Even though we had psychiatric curriculum as part of our training to be family doctors, most do not focus on psychiatric issues, since there are plenty of other medical problems and issues that we primary care doctors deal with on a daily basis. They may feel that psychiatry takes too much time, but I can assure you that this is simply not the case. I've been able to see the same number of patients that a typical family doctor sees while only focusing on primary care psychiatry, which I also refer to as mind-body medicine. I have devised a system that is easy to learn and understand, and a bonus is that it is also fun to do at the same time.

Most primary care doctors and many psychiatrists focus on symptomatic relief with what I label as "Band-Aid" solutions that focus on the symptoms but not the cause of the symptoms. Many primary care doctors treat low-grade depression and anxiety disorders but feel uncomfortable when an SSRI or other more basic medication doesn't work. They should at least switch to an SNRI and/or augment with Wellbutrin XL before then. Instead, they tend to refer to psychiatry for depression and anxiety, and definitely for bipolar disorder. Some primary care doctors don't think they see bipolar disorder, but I can assure them that they do. If they do recognize that, they may not want to be treated, but they should.

My hope, though, is that primary care providers play a much bigger role in helping these patients who are relying on us. We can easily learn how to get more comfortable treating these medical problems using breakthrough methods, using psychotropic medications to balance neurochemicals that are in need of being properly balanced in order to optimize mind-body health. My greatest hope and dream is that this book and my others will make a difference by helping primary care providers as well as specialists to learn The Corona Protocol and to use my methods in their practices.

This lack of recognition is unfortunately also the case with the majority of specialists, including pain specialists, who focus on a certain part of the body and treat disorders as they were trained to treat them, which makes sense. However, when it comes to neurochemical imbalances, that would probably not be a significant part of their training, so they don't tend to think in that fashion. Stress and mood are so related to every medical specialty; most doctors, even if they recognize the emotional-physical link, still don't treat these conditions in a neurochemically preventative way. They, like primary care doctors and psychiatrists, often tend to focus on symptom reduction and don't think outside of the box.

This symptom-based treatment approach may make patients happy, at least for the short term, since, of course, patients want their symptoms resolved that they went to the doctor for in the first place. They may resist this preventative approach by saying, "I don't want to take something daily; I only want to take something when I need to." It can be challenging to convince them that it's better to prevent symptoms in the first place rather than just treating them with symptomatic medications. They often end up taking the "band-aids" daily, which is contrary to their not wanting to take a medication daily. Pointing this out can sometimes help but sometimes doesn't.

The most popular "band-aid" medications are pain pills (opiate or non-opiate choices), anti-inflammatories, muscle relaxants, steroids (at times), minor tranquilizers (benzodiazepines), and sleeping pills. If there is a stress relation to whatever symptoms, these "band-aids" may work well in the short term and even in the long term; however, they don't really get to the underlying problem that caused the symptoms in the first place. There is also an addictive potential, as well as potential long-term side effects.

I prefer focusing on the underlying problems and fixing them while trying to minimize the symptomatic medications. Don't get me wrong. Symptomatic medications are still necessary and often an important part of the treatment, but they ideally should not be the focus. The more of them that are taken points out the need to get under the hood and figure out what is really going on and then fix it in the safest and most effective way.

The most common somatic symptoms that we deal with are headaches; neck/trapezius/shoulder/upper back pain (the most common); mid- to lower back pain; chest pain; TMJ/jaw pain from clenching and bruxism; IBS; and other stomach- and bowel-related symptoms such as acid reflux, abdominal cramping, bloating, diarrhea, constipation, etc. Fibromyalgia, dizziness and other neurological symptoms, hormonal symptoms, certain urinary symptoms, skin symptoms, cardiac symptoms, pulmonary symptoms, endocrine symptoms, and others.

Emotional and mood symptoms are also "real" medical diagnoses, such as anxiety disorders, depressive disorders, bipolar disorder, ADD/ADHD, eating disorders, OCD, PTSD, and many others, and are also very real to the person who is suffering. Other psychiatric conditions are often treated more with symptomatic medications than they are with preventative and curative psychotropic medications. As I said, patients expect relief of their symptoms, and it's quick and easy to just write a prescription and send them on their merry way.

It may take longer to explain to patients why preventative medications are better for them in the long run, and the time taken is certainly worth it. I refer to psychotropic medications as "holistic" since they work with the body to heal itself by balancing neurochemicals in the nervous system in a proper fashion only if they need to be balanced in the first place. We are then able to see the mind-body connection in action in order for our patients to feel their true selves again or for the first time.

What really started me down this road I have traveled was in the early 1990s, within a year of starting practice, when Effexor XR (venlafaxine ER) came out. Prior to that time, I had experience with the first three SSRIs: Prozac (fluoxetine), Zoloft (sertraline), and Paxil (paroxetine). I was amazed to see that with Effexor XR (venlafaxine ER), there was somatic symptom reduction as well as improved anxiety reduction at the same time.

I then figured out that was why the previous tricyclic antidepressants worked on not only mood but also somatic symptoms, though they were often not well tolerated. However, low doses then and now have been used to help sleep and somatic symptoms, due to the fact that there is dual action of balancing serotonin and norepinephrine with their use. That simple but profound discovery of the importance of norepinephrine is really what launched the new direction of my career and later writings.

The next important discovery regarding somatic symptoms was the role of GABA. I understood this early on with the use of gabapentin and Depakote, with which I saw anxiety reduction and improvement of mood and painful somatic symptoms all at the same time. I really became more interested, though, once I got experience prescribing Topamax (topiramate), which not only reduced pain and anxiety but also helped underlying mood, helped with addiction to alcohol and other drugs, and even helped people to lose weight, which is uncommon regarding psychotropic medications. I was already prescribing it "off-label" for migraine headaches way before the FDA approved it for that indication. I was also noticing many of the other symptomatic pain disorders previously mentioned were also responding to its use.

When I think of the reduction of somatic symptoms, I think of norepinephrine first and GABA second. However, sometimes it is the other way around. If I choose a GABA agent first, then I am probably suspecting the bipolar spectrum. An SNRI/GABAergic combination is a common "Dynamic Duo" in my practice for somatic and emotional complaints. Of course, serotonin, dopamine, and other factors may be involved, since when mood is improved by utilizing psychotropic medications in the ideal way, then the physical body can also respond favorably. If psychosomatic symptoms are not well controlled, then I do not consider that the patient is truly in full remission.

ADD/ADHD

If ADD/ADHD is a factor, then this also is important to address in order for patients to achieve maximal functioning. If the person has this along with a mood disorder, which happens all too frequently, it's important to treat them both at the same time. My tendency is to focus on stabilizing the mood first and getting rid of the depression, anxiety, and even hypomania and especially mania. In some cases, though, if the ADD/ADHD symptoms are prominent, then it may make sense to try treating that first, since this can also improve mood and lower anxiety at the same time. Stimulants tend to have a calming effect, providing calm and relaxed focus, as long as the dose is not raised too high. As a general rule, if stimulants increase anxiety, then the diagnosis is probably not ADD. Stimulants should calm the brain down. The other possibility is that the stimulant is uncovering bipolar disorder, which can be treated with a stimulant or non-stimulant ADD medication combined with one or more mood stabilizers.

What we often see is that when treating the mood disorder optimally, especially with an SNRI and/or Wellbutrin, we also may see resolution of ADD/ADHD symptoms. However, non-stimulants are often not enough when it comes to optimally treating ADD/ADHD, which usually requires a stimulant to achieve the best results. It typically just depends on the specific needs of the individual.

There are other potentially good choices to treat ADD/ADHD besides stimulants and certain antidepressants. Strattera (atomoxetine) is a NRI (norepinephrine reuptake inhibitor), with its main focus on norepinephrine but also a slight boosting effect on dopamine. The second NRI that was recently released at the time of this writing in 2025 is Qelbree (viloxazine), which focuses on norepinephrine but has a slight boosting effect on dopamine and even serotonin.

There are also two other non-stimulant medications used to treat ADD/ADHD: guanfacine and clonidine. I prefer the guanfacine ER version called Intuniv (guanfacine hydrochloride), which activates alpha 2a-adrenergic receptors in the brain. Clonidine has an alpha antagonistic effect on the brain and reduces sympathetic outflow. Both medications have a calming effect on the brain and tend to be sedating, which is why I dose them at bedtime since they can also help with sleep. The remaining effects are to reduce hyperactivity and impulsivity, which can both be related to ADD/ADHD, though the inattentive variation is more common. In my experience they don't seem to really treat the core ADD symptoms like stimulants do, and potentially the non-stimulants can be added to stimulants as an augmentation strategy.

Speaking of non-stimulants, there are other options that I mentioned. Provigil (modafinil) and Nuvigil (armodafinil) are basically dopamine reuptake inhibitors, with the newer Sunosi (solriamfetol) being a dopamine and norepinephrine reuptake inhibitor. This is why I often use Wellbutrin XL as an augmentation strategy, as well as SNRIs at times. We also have the two NRIs Strattera (atomoxetine) and Qelbree (viloxazine). Both of them boast of norepinephrine but also dopamine a bit, and Qelbree (viloxazine) also has a slight serotonin. Also, we can learn to be creative when it comes to the rational polypharmaceutical approach.

Problems with focus and concentration aren't always related to ADD. For example, it is not uncommon for those who are depressed to have these symptoms, as well as people with anxiety and bipolar disorder. For many patients just resolving the underlying mood disorder helps patients to focus and concentrate better, as well as have better energy and motivation. I find it interesting that antidepressants and mood stabilizers also might treat some of the core ADD symptoms at the same time. This is a win-win.

However, stimulants are not only the most efficacious treatment overall, but there are also potential side benefits. One of them can be suppression of appetite when needed, such as for those who "stress eat" with comfort foods and could benefit by the suppression of appetite as well as a boost to the metabolism. It also may boost energy so they are then more likely to start an exercise program and other healthy habits. We, of course, need to screen them properly to make sure that a stimulant is tolerated and safe as well as effective for the individual.

In order to optimally treat neurochemical imbalances, treating ADD may help to resolve mood symptoms that coexist with it. As I said, stimulants may actually lower anxiety and stress levels but can also boost the mood at the same time. If a stimulant increases anxiety, either the dose is too high, the wrong medication is being used, or the patient really does not have true ADD/ADHD. The patient's response to a stimulant helps us to confirm or deny this diagnosis. It also may uncover a different diagnosis not even previously considered.

Stimulants are not the only option when it comes to treating ADD/ADHD. Some providers are concerned that treating this runs the risk of destabilizing the mood. That is a valid concern, but if we know what we are doing, then we can learn how to balance and treat it in the safest and best way. By understanding how to treat mood and ADD at the same time, each can be a little tricky to balance but worth the effort to do so. If this occurs, it is much more likely that we will be able to provide patients with the best results imaginable. Stimulants also have the advantage of increasing energy, improving metabolism by helping with weight loss when needed, and improving depressive symptoms, including anxiety, and this results in an overall increase in functionality and an improved quality of life.

Some of the trickier types of patients are those with bipolar disorder and ADD at the same time. In these cases, it's important to make sure that the mood is adequately stabilized before addressing the ADD, but they can both be safely and effectively treated together. A concern may be that a stimulant will destabilize the mood, and thus some providers may hold back from treating ADD/ADHD because of that fear, but that really should not be a problem if they are both being treated correctly at the same time.

While treating the ADD, it's possible that we would need to increase one or more of the mood stabilizers to account for its addition, while in other cases that is not necessary. It also may be the case that mood stabilizers improve mood stability but worsen ADD symptoms, necessitating an increase in the stimulant dose. It is crucial then to fine-tune the stimulants and nonstimulants until they are perfectly balanced, or if we do not, then we may never reach remission in those cases. The different medication classes can be safely and effectively combined together, and if it is not optimally treated, then the patient will not be able to achieve true remission.

ADD is even more common with unipolar disorders, such as depression and anxiety disorders, and as I said previously, it is usually not the case that treating ADD worsens anxiety, but rather tends to reduce it. It's also the case that stimulants can be good augmenting agents with antidepressants since both diagnoses often coexist and can then be treated at the same time. Different classes of psychotropic medications, such as stimulants and nonstimulants, can work together in a symbiotic fashion.

A big misconception about ADD/ADHD is that it is only a childhood problem but not an adult problem. Even though the symptoms usually occur before the age of 12, most likely in early grade school, that does not mean that it cannot happen later. Many of these patients are highly intelligent and get by for a while with good work ethic, effort, and natural intelligence. However, for some in high school, college, and graduate school, or in a challenging work environment, the symptoms may become difficult for the person to manage.

Unfortunately, there are so many misperceptions about this subject among physicians, pharmacists, insurance companies, and many others who either do not think it is a real problem to begin with and think the person is just lazy or needs to try harder or believe it's only a childhood problem and that adults should be able to grow out of it. Some equate prescription stimulants with street "speed" and may say things such as, "You might as well just go on meth if you're going to take that crap." These views are uninformed, misinformed, ignorant, and just plain wrong, but unfortunately this is the case all too often. This "anti-pill" mentality is common and, in my opinion, is even an epidemic.

I have also seen that frequently pharmacists are ignorant about this condition and the role of stimulants and at times even shame those who are taking them. I think that they believe that all controlled substances are the same and that this is like the opiate crisis. The FDA/government is also misinformed about the proper treatment of ADD/ADHD. We need to learn how to combat this thinking by explaining in an easily understandable way how psychotropic medications work and why they are the best preventative and holistic solutions available.

Too often parents stand in the way of their children getting the help that they need because they take their advice from family and friends, the internet, and other similar ignorant opinions. They may say something like, "I was the same way when I was his or her age, and I turned out just fine." Some may take it as an insult to suggest that the child has a condition that at least one of the parents likely has. It certainly may be the case that certain patients outgrow at least some of the ADD symptoms when they get to adulthood with hard work and good organizational skills, but we should certainly not berate people or make them feel lesser than if they function their best with needed medical help.

Sometimes spouses, or friends and family, hold back adults from getting treatment by their negative comments and views, which can affect the person to the point that they may not be treated when they really should, due to unwarranted fears perpetuated by people who may mean well but are not helping the situation since they are not qualified to give medical advice. Even if the person is in a medical field, if that person is not trained to prescribe psychotropic medications, then their advice regarding medications should be ignored. I suggest to patients that they come to me for medical advice since that is my job.

It can be very frustrating when patients take the advice of others and not me. Other people have more access to them than I do, and that can have quite an effect when it comes to influencing patients' decisions. I stress to patients that these are very treatable conditions, and if they are not treated, then this will hold them back from achieving their true potential and happiest selves.

A controversial and tricky issue is what to do with the ADD/ADHD patient who has a history of addiction. Not all addictions are the same, so it doesn't mean that someone who has struggled with alcoholism, opiates, or others, should not receive a stimulant if needed for treatment of ADD/ADHD. If street stimulants, such as methamphetamines and cocaine, are not the addictive issue, this should not rule out treating ADD/ADHD with a controlled substance. Another sign of self-medicating is excessive consumption of power drinks, "energy" vitamins and supplements, and excessive caffeine intake.

Let's get even more controversial. Let's say the patient has a history of addiction to nonprescribed stimulants, such as cocaine, methamphetamines, or prescription stimulants acquired without a prescription. Many would opine that we should definitely avoid a stimulant, but I have found it to be appropriate in certain situations. Especially if the addiction is not recent and the patient has been in recovery, then that is an appropriate person to consider treatment.

The argument against would be that a prescribed stimulant would be a "gateway" drug back to the illegal variety. I have seen it happen that some people will abuse the stimulant that I give them, and in that case, I stop prescribing it. However, for many this is not the case, and they can take it as prescribed. They are certainly at higher-than-average risk, though, so it needs to be done carefully and thoughtfully, and the person needs to be monitored closely.

The other way of looking at it is that the patient may have been *self-medicating ADD*. One way to discern this is by taking a good history as to what the stimulant did for that person. Did the stimulant destabilize the mood, cause a speeding and racing of the brain, or lead to hypomania, mania, or somewhere in-between? This is where mood stabilizers would need to come into play before proceeding with caution.

Some patients are rational, while others are irrational, and if it is the latter and associated with psychotic thinking, then the stimulant certainly needs to be stopped, and the treatment plan needs to be reassessed. Once the patient is stabilized, in these cases we may want to then consider a non-stimulant option, though the stimulant is not out of the question in the right situation.

If the person previously had responded to a stimulant by not only improving focus and concentration but also by slowing the brain down and relaxing the patient, then this is probably a good candidate for treatment. If the person, though, doesn't really have ADD/ADHD, then the stimulant may be too activating and may potentially increase anxiety or worsen mood in general, and if that occurs, then we need to stop, reassess, and then redirect treatment in a different direction until we find the best solutions together.

Nonstimulants may be the preferred option for many doctors in higher-risk circumstances. They may work very well for some, but the reality is that in more patients than not, stimulants just work the best. These patients obviously need close monitoring, and if there is concern, we can do drug tests, check CURES reports, and monitor the prescriptions closely. The reality is that if we do not treat ADD/ADHD appropriately, these patients will self-medicate and treat themselves in ways that are not nearly as healthy. If ADD/ADHD is not treated optimally, then the person will not achieve true remission. We can show patients how full remission feels if we work together and treat the mind and body optimally at the same time.

Metabolic Changes/Lifestyle Habits

Even though metabolic issues may not be formal criteria for achieving remission, they are still, in my opinion, important to assess when it comes to overall mental and physical health. Increased or decreased appetite with significant weight gain or weight loss is one of the criteria for depression, so this issue is formally recognized. However, I feel that its importance is often underappreciated, since achieving remission is pursuing a higher quality of life, which is much more achievable if patients are healthy in their choices and behaviors. We can see how changes in mood can affect appetite in different ways.

If the patient is overeating and gaining an unhealthy level of weight, this is a form of "self-medicating" with "comfort foods" while "stress eating" in order to relieve depression and anxiety, even if just for the moment. This can be the case with food (especially sugars and carbohydrates), as it can for alcohol (liquid sugar and carbohydrates) and other drugs.

Other patients who are depressed and anxious tend to undereat and lose an unhealthy amount of weight, so different people respond differently when it comes to mood as it relates to appetite and change of weight. Symptoms related to mood, such as low motivation and low energy, apathy, and anhedonia, work against the person caring enough to change his or her routine by eating healthy and exercising regularly. If we optimally resolve the underlying mood disorders, then patients are more likely to make healthy choices for themselves with regard to eating habits and healthy lifestyle habits such as not smoking, not drinking too much, having a well-balanced diet, and maintaining a healthy and balanced exercise program.

Unhealthy choices regarding diet, exercise, and habits certainly occur in depressive and anxiety disorders, especially in bipolar disorder and schizophrenia. However, these choices are even more magnified when it comes to patients suffering with eating disorders. On one end of the spectrum, we have binge eating disorder and bulimia nervosa, both having to do with overeating, with the latter also involving voluntary elimination. They tend to crave sugars and carbohydrates (the binge foods) in particular, which temporarily relieves stress and provides comfort, however, when guilt and shame are then experienced, this leads to the process repeating itself over and over again. They do not have control over these behaviors because the underlying disorder actually ends up controlling them by laxative abuse, diuretics, or over-exercising, with the best known and "classic" behavior of voluntary purging. All of these have addictive components. For this reason, they are driven to provide themselves temporary soothing of their emotions. Unfortunately, though the relief is only temporary, they are driven to continue these unhealthy behaviors.

On the other end of the spectrum is anorexia nervosa, which is associated with a poor body image and body dysmorphia. They become addicted to withholding nutrition as a form of control and punishment, since in actuality they are being controlled internally by the disorder and want to feel some sense of power and control. The reality though, is that they end up being completely controlled and trapped in this way of thinking.

Bulimia and anorexic nervosa are among the most difficult disorders to treat, since there are so many different aspects and issues other than the neurochemical imbalances, such as personality type, upbringing, and relationships, as well as psychological, nutritional, and medical elements all at the same time. The team approach is the best for these patients in order to cover all our bases, including a nutritionist, a psychologist, and a physician or other practitioner who understands how to treat this most properly with so many terrific psychotropic medications that we are fortunate to be able to work with.

Whatever the diagnosis is that is affecting healthy lifestyle choices, thankfully there are some very effective psychotropic medications available to help patients combat these underlying urges. When it comes to depressive disorders as well as disordered eating, there is often a lack of motivation, energy, and drive to change. Wellbutrin XL (the bupropion form I prescribe the most), along with the newer name-brand Aplenzin, is a unique and amazing medication that is in a class by itself, since no other medication does what it does regarding blocking the reuptake of mostly dopamine and somewhat norepinephrine, thus creating a dopaminergic boost, which leads to its many benefits.

When patients are feeling better and are more motivated, then they are more likely to make healthy changes with regard to diet and exercise, as well as other habits. Wellbutrin also reduces the desire to smoke cigarettes, which is a useful asset. Wellbutrin is the second-best medication, along with nicotine replacement, when it comes to helping patients stop this very unhealthy habit. Chantix is the most effective, though, if you are not having success otherwise. Another potential benefit of Wellbutrin is appetite suppression, especially if that is needed and healthy for that person. Before prescribing Wellbutrin, though, it is important to make sure that the person with an eating disorder is medically stable and has had their lab work done, such as their electrolytes recently checked, to make sure they are stable enough.

The augmenting agent that I probably prescribe the second most after Wellbutrin XL is the unique medication Topamax (topiramate), which comes in a short-acting and three long-acting forms. Improving the flow of GABA in the nervous system results in a reduction of anxiety, improvement of mood, and reduction of pain and other somatic symptoms, as well as weight loss due to a reduction of the desire for sugars and carbohydrates. It may even decrease the desire for alcohol (liquid sugar and carbohydrates) and illicit drugs, such as marijuana and others. Thus, this medication improves lifestyle habits by putting the person more in control of the food choices and other lifestyle decision-making.[1]

Stimulants such as phentermine and ADD medications are also helpful by reducing appetite and thus reducing binge eating, as well as improving energy and motivation to change lifestyle habits. Stimulants also mix well with antidepressants and actually help to boost mood for some. Mixing and matching psychotropic medications should be the rule and not the exception. There are many other psychotropic medications that are weight-neutral or more likely to cause weight gain, so it is nice to have a few choices that do the opposite. Some-

1 For a much more extensive discussion about Eating Disorders check out chapter 12 entitled "Eaten Alive by Eating Disorders" in my first book of the *Healing the Mind and Body* trilogy series.

times I add Topamax (topiramate) just for its weight loss benefit, especially if the medication that is causing some weight gain is working well for the patient, and thus, I don't want to remove it. Psychotropic medications such as these help patients to be more in control of their decision-making.

Overeating and overindulging in any way with resultant weight gain and difficulty losing it is a more common problem than undereating and losing too much weight. Just improving the underlying mood disorder may be enough to encourage healthier eating habits by using whichever medications are needed in order to achieve healthier eating habits. The correct psychotropic medications can help the person be more in control and thus make healthier choices. The optimal combination of psychotropic medications needed is worth the time it takes to get the mix right and achieve the ultimate goal of full and complete remission.

In some patients increasing appetite is a good thing, as long as the person is mentally able to deal with the weight gain, which in the case of anorexia nervosa does not come easily. In these cases, hopefully when the mood is actually improved, then the patient will be able to mentally deal with weight gain that is desperately needed for one's health. Certain antidepressants may cause weight gain, but for the most part they are weight-neutral. However, if a medication works very well but leads to weight gain, then we can focus on lifestyle habits, and if needed, we can add a medication that promotes weight loss, such as Topamax (topiramate), Wellbutrin, and/or a stimulant. Putting together the proper psychotropic medications with the rational polypharmaceutical approach is the healthiest, nonaddictive, and preventative way to deal with mind-body imbalances.

The medication class that is best known for weight gain is the atypical antipsychotics. Some cause more and some cause less, so what to use depends on the situation. If the patient really needs to gain weight, then Zyprexa (olanzapine) or one of the others that increase appetite may be a good choice. It is also possible that once adequate weight is gained, then the medication can be switched to another in this class that is less likely to continue this trend, such as Latuda, Geodon (ziprasidone), Vraylar (cariprazine), Caplyta (lumateperone), Lybalvi (olanzapine and samidorphan), or Fanapt (iloperidone). Atypicals are a very important class for treating difficult disorders such as eating disorders and challenging cases of depression and anxiety. These patients often have an underlying bipolar spectrum disorder, and their treatment most likely requires a combination of antidepressants and mood stabilizers. This follows the rational trial-and-error method I have devised.

True remission goes well beyond just the HAM-D score. Having a good metabolism and being at a healthy weight may not be part of the formal criteria for remission, but I look at this as well as all of the other factors before I consider the outcome to be a success. We need to work closely with each patient in order to address their concerns and achieve their desires, with the goal being a happy and healthy life, also known as full and complete remission, for as many as humanly possible.

Residual Symptoms

When remission is discussed, we are usually referring to depression; however, I think of remission as a broader term that relates to any psychiatric and psychosomatic diagnosis. If we treat the "primary" diagnosis to resolution, but then we uncover other diagnoses, then we need to shift our focus to treating those also. For example, if we are treating depression but then we also uncover ADD, an anxiety disorder, bipolar spectrum symptoms, or others, then we need to shift our focus to dealing with the other conditions as well. We can develop a feel for treating coexisting conditions in the proper order. If we treat bipolar disorder or other mood disorders but then have residual ADD or other mood symptoms, then we need to keep treating until all issues are resolved.

The point is that most psychiatric conditions do not travel alone. There are many potential residual symptoms that are not necessarily thought about when we're focusing on treating the diagnosis at hand. Symptoms, such as decreased sex drive or sexual functioning, insomnia, fatigue, poor focus and concentration, anhedonia, nervous habits, and many other symptoms, are in need of attention. So many people are suffering unnecessarily, and that needs to change.

I always record a full review of systems and symptoms at the first visit and then every visit thereafter, since we need to constantly make sure that all relevant symptoms are being addressed properly. We often cannot take care of them all at once, so we need to prioritize which are the most important to address first and what can wait until later.

I try to notice if more than one symptom can be treated at one time in order to "kill two birds with one stone," such as switching from an SSRI to an SNRI to treat somatic symptoms along with anxiety and other mood symptoms. Adding Wellbutrin can not only resolve sexual side effects, improve energy and motivation, and boost mood but also improve ADD symptoms, such as focus and concentration, as well as executive functioning and even memory. I may consider Topamax (topiramate) to deal with not only anxiety and somatic symptoms such as headaches and others but also to help people lose weight and cut down on drinking and illicit drug use.

I may use a mood stabilizer not only to reduce mania and hypomania but also to stop mood cycling, depression, anxiety disorders, and other mood-related problems. We need to be open to augmenting as much as necessary to achieve the goal of full and complete remission. This means recognizing not only depression and anxiety but also the subtle signs of the bipolar spectrum, requiring a mixture of antidepressants and mood stabilizers in order to find the best recipe with the most satisfying results.

If somatic symptoms are still present and related to neurochemical imbalances, then I keep trying until they are resolved for good. Even when we reach remission, that does not mean our work is done. We need to make sure that we monitor them closely and carefully in order to keep them there.

They may be doing great, but then a few months later, or six or more months, or even a year or more later, they may fall back into a cyclical pattern of somatic symptoms, depression, anxiety, or mood destabilization. This means we need to reassess whether what is being taken needs to be changed or if we simply need to augment, such as with a different antidepressant, with the antidepressant/mood stabilizer Lamictal (lamotrigine), or with a different mood stabilizer altogether.

Our goal is not only to get people to full remission by resolving the symptoms that had plagued the person and lowered that individual's quality of life. It is also important to make sure they stay that way for good by being able to stay optimally balanced in full and complete remission and mind-body harmony over the long haul.

Notes

Notes

Notes

Notes

OTHER BOOKS BY PAUL D. CORONA, M.D.

Healing the Mind and Body: The Trilogy

Healing the Mind and Body: Volume 1, Second Edition

Healing the Mind and Body: Volume 2, Second Edition

Healing the Mind and Body: The Doctor and Patient Guide, *Volume 3, Second Edition.*

The Corona Protocol Three Secrets to Success

The Corona Protocol Prescriber's Guide

The Corona Protocol: *A Scientifically Proven Medical Solution to STOP Addiction, Bullying, Homelessness, School Shootings and Suicide. 30 years in the making*